Safe Harbor

Navigating the Depths of Trauma with Informed Therapy

by
Well-Being Publishing

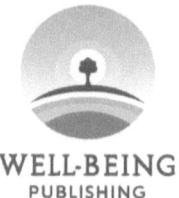

To You,

Thank you!

Table of Contents

Introduction:
Embracing Trauma-Informed Care

In the increasingly complex field of mental health, trauma-informed care has emerged as a beacon of empathy and effectiveness, guiding us toward a deeper understanding of the intricate tapestry of human experience. As mental health professionals, we bear witness to the harsh realities of psychological trauma and its profound impact on the lives of those we serve. Embracing trauma-informed care is not merely an intellectual exercise; it is a heartfelt commitment to validating and healing the wounds of the past. In this pursuit, we strive to foster environments that not only acknowledge the pervasiveness of trauma but also champion resilience and recovery.

At the heart of trauma-informed care lies the undeniable truth that trauma is pervasive, and its tendrils can touch anyone, regardless of age, ethnicity, or social standing. The journey to healing is personal and laden with challenges. Yet, every step taken is a testament to the human spirit's capacity to rise above adversity. As clinicians, therapists, and counselors, we're tasked with the sacred duty of joining our clients on this arduous yet noble journey, equipped with the knowledge and compassion that can light the way.

Understanding trauma means delving into the quagmire of the human psyche, unraveling the sheer force of events that can change the course of a life. It means recognizing that each person's experience with trauma is unique, and their narrative is not simply a collection of symptoms but a story that deserves to be heard and honored. It is within this narrative that we find the keys to unlock the paths to recovery.

Implementing trauma-informed care is a transformative practice that demands we move beyond traditional therapeutic boundaries. It calls for a paradigm shift where respect, safety, and collaboration become the cornerstones of our approach, fostering an atmosphere where individuals feel seen, heard, and empowered. As we marvel at the resilience reflected in those who seek our help, we must continually refine our methods and strategies, so they resonate with empathy and promote healing.

What drives us toward trauma-informed care is not only a tapestry of theories and methodologies but the profound human connection at its core. To bear witness to another's pain, to sit alongside them in their darkest moments, to gently nurture hope when it feels most elusive—these are the acts that define our work.

Our roles as practitioners weave us into the very fabric of our clients' journeys. As we delve into this book, we acknowledge our responsibility to provide a sanctuary of safety—a place where life stories can be shared without fear of judgment. The therapeutic relationship is our vessel through which healing waters can flow. In this sanctuary, empowerment is more than an abstract concept. It is a palpable force that fuels recovery and reclamation of agency.

The subsequent chapters will guide us through a comprehensive exploration of trauma—the multifaceted impact it has on mind and body, the principles that shape our therapeutic engagements, and the foundational approaches that underpin our practice. We delve into specific strategies, from somatic methods that address the preverbal echoes of distress to narrative techniques that rewrite the scripts of survivors. Each chapter builds upon the next, creating a holistic framework for trauma-informed care that is both theoretically sound and practically applicable.

As we embrace trauma-informed care, we celebrate the diversity of human experience. Assessing and tailoring our approaches to each individual's needs requires cultural sensitivity and an unwavering belief in the dignity of all persons. As we navigate through attachment theory, somatic approaches, and cognitive-behavioral interventions, our minds remain open to the endless possibilities of healing and growth.

We recognize that advances in trauma therapy are constantly evolving. Standing at the forefront of emerging research and integrative techniques, we commit to being lifelong learners in a field as dynamic as it is rewarding. Our call to action extends beyond the individual to groups, communities, and systemic structures that all play a crucial role in supporting recovery from trauma. The power of connection—within therapy groups, through community support and beyond—becomes a healing balm for the isolated pain of trauma.

Special population segments hold unique stories and challenges, urging us to broaden our lens and to diversify our strategies to honor every individual's lived experience. Whether working with children, older adults, or marginalized groups, we hold space for the manifold expressions of trauma and recovery, always remaining responsive to the nuances presented by each person's life stage and social context.

Interdisciplinary collaboration is also imperative, as the interactions between pharmacological interventions and psycho-therapeutic techniques carry transformative potential. Navigating this landscape with wisdom and integrity, we build bridges with allied professionals to provide the most comprehensive care possible.

In the course of our practice, the need for self-care becomes an essential narrative in itself. We acknowledge the weight of vicarious trauma and recognize the essential practice of nurturing our own well-being as clinicians. Only then can we sustain the ability to bring our fullest presence to those in need. We must be vigilant in tending to our own hearts, minds, and spirits to continue serving as pillars of strength for those embarking on healing journeys.

The future of trauma therapy shines bright with promise. From technological advancements to advocacy efforts that shape policy, we stand on the cusp of a new era—an era where trauma-informed care is not just an option but a standard that permeates the very essence of mental health services. Every innovation, every piece of research, every shared story propels us forward in our quest to understand, alleviate, and ultimately transform the impact of trauma.

In this introduction, we stand together at the threshold of discovery, poised to explore the expansive realm of trauma-informed care. Let this book be a companion on your professional journey, a source of inspiration, and a reminder that in the space between brokenness and healing lies our ability to effect change. As practitioners, our task is to embrace the mantle of trauma-informed care with humility and courage, ever committed to the betterment of those we serve and the enrichment of the therapeutic practice at large.

Chapter 1:
Understanding Trauma

Embarking on the journey of trauma-informed care requires a keen awareness that every individual's experience is inherently unique, paving the path for a strong empathetic foundation from which healing can begin. Within the tapestry of human experience, traumatic events stand out for their profound impact on a person's mental, emotional, and physical wellbeing. The essence of understanding trauma lies not just in recognizing its visible aftermath but in comprehending the complex interplay between environmental variables and the individual's neurobiological makeup. From the sudden shock of acute trauma to the deep-rooted scars of chronic experiences, the diverse nature of trauma influences each survivor in a multitude of ways, giving shape to the necessity of tailor-made therapeutic frameworks. As we delve into the profound ways in which trauma can influence the mind and body, it becomes evident that the nuances of each person's experience demand more than a textbook approach; they call for an integrative, dynamic, and compassionate strategy to facilitate a journey of resiliency and recovery. Recognizing the vast spectrum of traumatic experiences, from single incidents to pervasive and complex patterns, empowers mental health professionals to construct a solid groundwork for therapy that respects the delicate balance between strength and vulnerability inherent in every survivor.

The intricate nature of traumatic experiences is as diverse as the individuals who endure them. It is crucial to grasp the complexity and variability inherent in trauma to better serve those seeking restoration and resilience through therapy. In this segment, we delve deeply into the nature of traumatic experiences, laying the foundation for a more profound comprehension of its impacts on the human psyche and body.

Trauma is an emotional response to profoundly distressing or disturbing events that overwhelm an individual's capacity to cope, causing feelings of helplessness, diminishing their sense of self and their ability to feel a full range of emotions and experiences. Traumatic events can defy the ordinary and push the boundaries of what individuals perceive as predictable and controllable in their world.

It is important to recognize the subjective nature of trauma; what might be traumatic for one person may not be for another. This subjectivity is rooted in an individual's life history, psychological constitution, and the presence of support systems, among other factors. Such relativity does not diminish the validity of one's traumatic experience but rather highlights the personal lens through which it is perceived and processed.

Trauma can erupt suddenly, as in natural disasters or accidents, or it can accumulate quietly over time, as in cases of prolonged neglect or chronic maltreatment. The singular moments of agony live side by side with protracted periods of anxiety, and both can profoundly challenge individuals' well-being and functioning.

Traumatic experiences often defy verbal articulation. They can consume an individual with their intensity, leaving their conscious mind grappling with confusion and disbelief. The horror can be so severe that the mind enlists defense mechanisms, such as dissociation, to safeguard the individual from the full impact of the trauma at the moment it occurs.

Encounters with trauma frequently produce a sense of disconn-ection— from oneself, others, and the wider world. This disconnection can manifest as detachment from emotions or as a disassociation from the physical body, leading to a fragmented feeling of existence. Recognition of this sense of disconnection is paramount in guiding individuals through the healing journey.

Responses to trauma can appear immediately or may be delayed, sometimes surfacing only weeks, months, or even years later. This latency can complicate the healing process, as the connection between the traumatic event and the emotional response may not be immediately obvious. For mental health professionals, understanding the ebb and flow of traumatic responses is essential when navigating the tides of recovery.

Survivors of trauma frequently grapple with intense feelings of guilt, shame, and self-blame. Revisiting and restructuring these emotions through therapy is not only transformative but also necessary for healing. The therapeutic space must allow for the safe exploration of these intense emotions.

Resilience in the face of trauma is not an innate trait but a complex interplay of variables including genetics, personal history, and environmental factors. While some individuals demonstrate remarkable fortitude, others might require more support to foster resilience. This variability emphasizes the need for individualized therapeutic interventions.

Among the most insidious aspects of trauma is the way it can become a lens through which survivors interpret the world, often distorting their perceptions and expectations. Reality, through a trauma-affected prism, can become hostile or unpredictable, shaping one's cognitive schema in long-lasting ways.

The ripples of trauma can extend beyond the individual, affecting families, communities, and cultures. Transgenerational trauma, for instance, is a critical consideration, where the effects of traumatic experiences are passed down and influence the subsequent generations. This broader context must not be overlooked, as it can play a pivotal role in an individual's experience and recovery from trauma.

Therapeutic work with trauma survivors is a profound responsebility that involves building trust, fostering a safe therapeutic environment, and carefully navigating the complexities of traumatic recall and reprocessing. It is an endeavor that requires not only professional aptitude but also an empathetic heart.

The transformative potential of therapy for those who have experienced trauma is profound. The therapeutic journey can reframe narratives of helplessness into stories of survival and growth, allowing the reclamation of one's agency and the rewriting of one's life story.

As practitioners, it is imperative to approach each individual's traumatic experience with sensitivity, acknowledging its unique nature while drawing from a broad spectrum of therapeutic methods. In doing so, we honor both the commonalities and the distinctiveness of the traumatic experience, facilitating a pathway to healing that is as informed as it is compassionate.

In essence, understanding the nature of traumatic experiences requires a nuanced approach that respects the multifaceted reality of trauma. It is a balance of science and soul that can lead to healing and the rediscovery of wholeness for those we serve. As we move forward, we shall delve deeper into the impact of trauma on the mind and body and explore the ways in which we can support individuals in their courageous journeys toward recovery.

The Impact of Trauma on the Mind and Body

As we traverse the landscape of understanding trauma, it's imperative to recognize its profound impact on both the mind and body. Trauma, akin to an unwelcome intruder, disrupts the equilibrium of our mental and physical states, leaving behind a complex web of challenges that we, as healers and guides, must address with the utmost care. The tendrils of trauma reach deep, entangling the nervous system, skewing perception, and barricading the potential for growth and healing. It is as if trauma speaks a language that pervades the psyche, sometimes silencing the voice of reason and other times amplifying fears to deafening volumes. Conversely, the body, in its resilience, bears the burdens of unspeakable experiences, often manifesting symptoms that are as tangible as they are symbolic. These symptoms serve as both a testament to the body's desire to communicate what the mind cannot express and a barrier to reintegration of self. In this way, understanding the symbiotic relationship between mind and body in the aftermath of trauma becomes a cornerstone of our therapeutic journey, paving the way for holistic healing and the reclamation of empowerment that is the birthright of every individual we have the honor to support.

Neurobiological Effects of Trauma

In our endeavor to illuminate the path towards healing, it is pivotal to grasp the profound neurobiological effects of trauma on the human body. A comprehensive understanding of these effects equips mental health professionals with the ability to tailor interventions that resonate with the complex needs of those who have experienced trauma. Through exploring the myriad ways that trauma can alter neurobiology, we stand on the cusp of fostering deeper empathy and more effective therapeutic strategies. As we delve into the intricacies of the brain's response to distressing events, we see a tapestry of neural activity that reveals much about our capacity for resilience and recovery.

At the core of traumatic responses lies the brain's alarm system, the amygdala, which becomes highly activated during traumatic events. This heightened state can lead to an oversensitivity to perceived threats, long after the trauma has passed. The amygdala's interaction with the prefrontal cortex, the center for executive functions such as decision-making and impulse control, is often compromised. This can result in diffculties with emotional regulation and an impaired ability to manage stress.

The body's natural stress response is regulated by the hypothalamic-pituitary-adrenal (HPA) axis. Trauma can dysregulate this system, causing an imbalance in stress hormone levels such as cortisol and adrenaline. These hormonal fluctuations can lead to chronic stress, which unnervingly alters both physical and mental health.

Neuroimaging studies have shown that trauma can actually change the structure and function of the brain. Areas such as the hippo-campus, which is vital for memory consolidation, can become atrophied after prolonged exposure to stress. This shrinking of the hippocampus may lead to impairments in forming new memories and accessing old ones, a common struggle among those with trauma histories.

The interconnectedness of the brain means that the impact of trauma is not localized to one area. Changes in one system often influence others, creating a ripple effect that can alter perception, cognition, and behavior. For instance, trauma can affect the salience network, which is responsible for determining what stimuli are important and deserve attention, leading to hypervigilance or difficulty concentrating.

Trauma also manifests in the body's sensory systems. The nervous system can become 'stuck' in a state of hyperarousal, comparable to an alarm that doesn't shut off, leading to symptoms like insomnia, irritability, and an exaggerated startle response. Conversely, there can be a numbing effect, wherein an individual feels detached from their surroundings and themselves, known as hypoarousal.

Understanding how trauma imprints itself on the nervous system elucidates why somatic symptoms are so prevalent. Individuals may experience chronic pain, gastrointestinal issues, and other somatic complaints that mystify medical professionals, without the realization that these are tethered to traumatic stress.

Neuroplasticity, the brain's ability to reorganize itself by forming new neural connections throughout life, offers a glimmer of hope. It is this very plasticity that enables healing from trauma to be a feasible goal. Therapeutic interventions, such as mindfulness and meditation, have been shown to promote positive changes in brain structure and function, contributing to the recovery process.

Oxytocin, sometimes dubbed the 'love hormone', is also implicated in the trauma response. This neurotransmitter, known for its role in social bonding and trust, can become dysregulated, affecting an individual's capacity to form and maintain healthy relationships after trauma.

The neurobiological effects of trauma underscore the importance of adopting a trauma-informed approach in therapy. It's crucial that treatments aren't just about discussing traumatic events, but also about recognizing and addressing the embodied nature of trauma. Integrating modalities that directly impact the nervous system to reestablish a sense of safety and regulation is essential for holistic healing.

The lens through which we view neurobiology should reflect a balance of understanding the challenges and harnessing the potential for change. Trauma can lead to neurobiological alterations that present formidable obstacles, yet it is within the inherent malleability of the brain that we find the seeds of transformation.

In our therapeutic work, acknowledging the biological underpinnings of trauma enables us to work with the body, not against it. It calls for us to be innovative, integrating practices that honor both the mind and the body, as we guide individuals on their journey towards health and restoration.

Neurobiological insights also open avenues for collaboration with other professionals, such as psychiatrists and neurologists, to create comprehensive care plans. It's important to consider the possibility of pharmacological interventions that can complement psychotherapy by alleviating some of the neurochemical imbalances caused by trauma.

Ultimately, the neurobiological effects of trauma challenge us to expand our therapeutic horizons. We're encouraged to not only consider the story of what happened but to also craft a narrative of recovery that includes reconnection with one's body and mind. The goal is to empower individuals to develop skills and strategies that bolster resilience and foster an enduring sense of safety within themselves.

In the next segments, we'll explore the psychological repercussions of trauma, reflecting on how these interplay with the neurobiological aspects we've discussed. It is within the synthesis of these under-standings that we can craft therapeutic interventions that resonate with the full spectrum of an individual's experience after trauma.

Psychological Repercussions of Trauma

In our journey of comprehending trauma and its profound impacts, we venture into the realm of the mind, contemplating the psychological aftereffects that trauma imprints upon individuals. The ripple effects of traumatic experiences are vast and nuanced, touching on cognitive, emotional, and social dimensions of a person's world. Through the lens of a therapist, one must hold space for this multifaceted metamorphosis of the psyche post-trauma.

When trauma occurs, it disrupts the narrative of one's life, creating incongruence between past understandings and present experiences. This dissonance may manifest as cognitive confusion, where beliefs and thoughts are challenged, often leading to pervasive self-doubt and questioning of reality. The therapist's role, then, is to illuminate pathways that reconcile these fragments, weaving a new tapestry of meaning.

Emotionally, trauma can unleash a tempest within, leading to complex reactions like anxiety, depression, and anger. These emotional responses, though they may seem unsettling, are natural reactions to unnatural events. In the therapeutic space, we validate these emotions, understanding them as signals, as messages from the psyche that need to be heard and acknowledged with compassion.

At the core of the psychological repercussions of trauma lies post-traumatic stress disorder (PTSD), a condition with symptoms that can hold a tight grip on an individual's daily functioning. The echoes of the past continue to haunt through flashbacks, nightmares, and an exaggerated startle response. Treatment must focus on helping individuals regain a sense of control and rebuild the trust in their personal narrative.

The avoidance of trauma reminders is a common and understandable response, but one that reinforces the walls of isolation and hinders recovery. Therapy seeks to gently dismantle these barriers, encouraging engagement with life and the reclamation of joy and purpose through paced and sensitive exposure.

Another psychological repercussion is the alteration in perceptions of threat. A traumatized individual can develop an altered threat perception, seeing danger where it does not exist, leading to hypervigilance and an exhausting state of constant alertness. Our therapeutic intervention can introduce a sense of safety and recalibrate these misattuned alarm systems.

Dissociation, a sophisticated defense mechanism, serves as an escape from the immediacy of trauma but can persist as a maladaptive separation from reality. Clients might describe feeling disconnected from their bodies, their emotions, or even their sense of self. In therapy, we strive to integrate these dissociated aspects for holistic healing.

Moreover, interpersonal relationships profoundly suffer under the weight of trauma. It's not uncommon for survivors to experience difficulties in trust, intimacy, and social engagement. As therapists, we aim to not only repair these relational wounds but also empower clients to forge stronger, more authentic connections with others.

Furthermore, one's self-concept and identity can be drastically reshaped by traumatic experiences. Often, victims of trauma can internalize a damaged self-narrative, feeling irreversibly broken or unworthy. Through therapeutic partnerships, one can confront these self-limiting beliefs, gradually reconstructing a strengthened identity that honors both their resilience and vulnerability.

When considering psychological repercussions, we cannot over-look the maladaptive coping strategies that emerge, such as substance abuse or self-harm. These strategies represent attempts to manage unbearable pain and symptoms, yet they compound distress. By acknowledging the underlying pain and fostering healthier coping mechanisms, therapy promotes sustainable healing.

Anxiety disorders beyond PTSD, such as generalized anxiety disorder and panic disorder, may emerge or be exacerbated by trauma. These can limit a person's ability to function and enjoy life. Through targeted approaches, we can help clients navigate these anxiety landscapes, ultimately retuning the nervous system to a more balanced state.

Mood disruptions are another chapter in the psychological repertoire of trauma's aftermath, where survivors might swing between emotional highs and lows, or find themselves in the grips of a persistent depressive state. It's a testament to the profound effect trauma has on the emotional brain, necessitating therapeutic strategies that address these mood dysregulations.

In the shadows of trauma resides a deep sense of shame and guilt, emotions that can become consuming in the aftermath of traumatic events. These feelings may revolve around what one did or didn't do during the event, or the belief that one is bad or wrong because of what happened. Healing in therapy involves addressing these corrosive emotions, fostering a renewed sense of self-acceptance and forgiveness.

Thus, the psychological repercussions of trauma are far-reaching, touching every corner of a person's existence. In therapy, we guide individuals through the transformation of their traumatic experiences, not aiming to forget or erase, but to understand and integrate these parts into a stronger whole. This journey requires patience, persistence, and a deep sense of hope, and as therapists, we walk alongside clients on this path of recovery, bearing witness to their ability to overcome and grow beyond their trauma.

As we progress through our exploration, the multifaceted nature of psychological trauma continues to be illuminated. Bearing witness to the journey of trauma survivors injects a profound sense of purpose into our work as therapists. The process of healing is an art, interweaving the threads of clinical knowledge with the humanity of each individual, creating a mosaic of recovery that respects the uniqueness of every trauma narrative.

Types of Trauma and Their Distinctions

As we delve deeper into the complex labyrinth of trauma, it's imperative to discern the nuances among the various forms of trauma individuals may encounter. Acute trauma arises from a single, distressing event, searing itself into the psyche with its immediate impact. In contrast, chronic trauma is the result of repeated and prolonged exposure to distressing experiences, often leading to a deep-rooted sense of insecurity and mistrust. Then there's complex trauma, which stems from diverse and multiple traumatic events, often occurring within the context of interpersonal relationships. This intricate tapestry of pain can lead to multi-faceted symptoms that challenge even the most experienced therapists. Understanding these distinct types, alongside their idiosyncratic manifestations and consequences, empowers mental health professionals to tailor their therapeutic approaches with precision, empathy, and effectiveness, thereby lighting the path toward healing and transformation for their clients.

Acute, Chronic, and Complex Trauma

Understanding the distinctions between acute, chronic, and complex trauma is central to effectively supporting those we aim to help heal. As mental health professionals, our grasp of these concepts forms the bedrock of trauma-informed care. Acute trauma typically follows a single, distressing event, often leaving individuals reeling from the sudden impact on their psychological well-being. The human spirit, while resilient, can be profoundly shaken by such occurrences, and our therapeutic approaches must be attuned to the nuances of these disruptions.

Chronic trauma, on the other hand, refers to repeated and prolonged exposure to stressful or harmful events. This could stem from situations such as enduring abuse, living in a war-torn area, or any environment where trauma is a constant, lurking presence. Here, the challenge is not just addressing a singular event, but rather a series of traumas that have potential to become deeply woven into an individual's psyche, reflecting patterns that may shape responses to stress and relationships for years to come.

Complex trauma is perhaps the most demanding to address, as it entails both the chronic nature of exposure to adverse events and the significant impact on a person's development. Often rooted in early life experiences, complex trauma can fundamentally affect a person's sense of self, their ability to form secure attachments, and their perception of safety in the world. As caregivers, recognizing the pervasive influence of complex trauma is essential in fostering an atmosphere of deep understanding and support.

When encountering acute trauma in a therapeutic setting, it is vital to establish safety and stabilize emotions. The immediate aftermath of a traumatic event leaves individuals in a heightened state of arousal. This stage is about grounding and reassuring the person that they are secure and supported in the present moment, allowing for the initial processing of their experiences.

Managing chronic trauma requires a different approach. Here, themes of trust, consistency, and predictability take on heightened importance. Clients may have ingrained coping mechanisms or beliefs that have served them in their repeated encounters with trauma. Unpacking and reshaping these aspects without judgment is critical if we are to help our clients rebuild their understanding of stability and predictability.

Complex trauma involves integrating various therapeutic modalities tailored to address not just the experiences of trauma themselves, but their wide-ranging effects on a person's life. A key focus is on reconstructing a sense of identity that has been compromised or fragmented by ongoing traumatic events. The work is often long-term and requires a steadfast commitment from both the practitioner and the client.

Understanding the neurobiological impacts of different trauma types informs our therapeutic efforts. For acute trauma, swift intervention can prevent the consolidation of traumatic memories in a way that leads to chronic symptoms. With chronic trauma, we are often dealing with ingrained neural pathways that need re-shaping and a body that has been conditioned to live in a state of constant alert. In complex trauma, the practitioner must be sensitive to the likelihood of pervasive developmental changes and a potential range of adaptive behaviors that have been adopted for survival.

The markers of effective therapy in treating trauma of all kinds include creating a safe therapeutic environment, instilling hope, and empowering the individual. This is particularly challenging when a client's history of trauma has eroded their sense of safety and trust in the world and in themselves. As healers, we must offer a reliable presence that can help counterbalance their experiences of unpredictability and chaos.

Cultural competency also plays a critical role in addressing trauma. Different cultures may have distinct ways of expressing and interpreting the experience of trauma. Our ability to contextualize and respect these differences is key to providing support that is not only effective but also honors the individuality of each client's background.

In the light of chronic and complex trauma, where an individual's narrative may be fragmented or riddled with gaps, we must also be skilled listeners. The art of narrative reconstruction can play a pivotal role in healing, allowing individuals to regain a sense of agency over their story. Storytelling can be a powerful tool, as it helps individuals process and integrate traumatic experiences into their overall life context.

Research continues to evolve in our understanding of trauma and its effects. Staying abreast of current findings and integrating them into practice enhances our ability to serve our clients effectively.

Innovations such as trauma-focused cognitive-behavioral therapy, eye movement desensitization and reprocessing (EMDR), and somatic experiencing provide an array of tools to address the multifaceted nature of trauma.

The concept of post-traumatic growth is also essential to explore within the realms of acute, chronic, and complex trauma. While acknowledging the profound pain and struggle that trauma brings, it is just as vital to recognize the potential for individuals to emerge with new strengths, deeper insights, and an enriched perspective on life. Instilling hope is not a naive act; it is a fundamental part of the healing process.

In the realms of chronic and complex trauma, self-care for the therapist is not an indulgence; it is a professional necessity. The work is demanding, and the risk of vicarious traumatization is high. To sustain the capacity to provide hope and healing, therapists themselves need strategies to replenish and safeguard their well-being.

Finally, the journey through trauma therapy is not a linear path. It can be filled with unexpected setbacks and breakthroughs. What remains constant, however, is the need for compassion, patience, and a deep belief in the human capacity for resilience. As practitioners, we are tasked with holding a therapeutic space that is both reflective and dynamic, one that honors the deeply personal and sometimes harrowing journey of recovery from trauma. Through our own dedication and growth as therapists, we cultivate the possibility of transformation for those who entrust us with their most vulnerable selves.

Chapter 2:
Foundations of Trauma-Informed Therapy

As we delve into the bedrock of trauma-informed therapy, it becomes clear that our approach can't simply mirror a traditional clinical framework; it must be a sanctuary for healing. In these foundations lie the cornerstones of compassionate care: principles that guide us to engage with clients not just as clinicians, but as guardians of a safe therapeutic space where trust can take root. Together, we build a clinician-client rapport anchored in an unwavering commitment to safety, respect, and collaboration. It is in this collaborative endeavor that we lay down the empowering groundwork, steering clear of retraumatization and championing a client's autonomy. Imagine a therapy room as a nurturing soil, where through understanding and consistent care, the most fragile beginnings of recovery can burgeon into resilient growth.

Principles of a Trauma-Informed Approach

An effective trauma-informed approach rests on a solid understanding of the principles that anchor it. These guiding tenets shape our interactions with clients, informing every aspect of therapy to create a supportive healing environment. These principles aren't just theoretical concepts; they represent a concrete commitment to understanding, acknowledging, and responding to the impacts of trauma.

Safety, both physical and emotional, stands at the forefront of trauma-informed care. Therapists must cultivate an environment where clients feel secure to explore their most painful memories. This safe space is not born out of chance; it is meticulously created and maintained through consistent, predictable actions and a sensitive therapy process that prioritizes the client's sense of control and well-being.

Trustworthiness is crucial in building the therapeutic relationship. Transparency in practice, including clear explanations about the therapy process and consistency in behavior, lays a foundation for trust. With trust, you can forge a path together with your clients, a path that's aligned with healing and growth.

Trauma survivors often feel a profound loss of control and power in their lives. A trauma-informed approach emphasizes collaboration, inviting clients to become active participants in their healing journey. This collaborative stance honors the individual's autonomy and fosters empowerment in decision-making and goal-setting.

Peer support, often an undervalued aspect of healing, is an integral part of a trauma-informed framework. It provides clients with a sense of belonging and connection, which can be transformative. Incorporating peer perspectives and experiences can help demonstrate the possibility of recovery and build a community of healing.

Another pillar of trauma-informed care is the acknowledgment of cultural, historical, and gender issues. It encompasses a deep respect for the client's background and identity, and a responsive approach that is mindful of social contexts, prejudices, and systemic inequalities that may influence the client's experiences.

Off the back of these principles, it's important not to overlook the concept of 'voice and choice.' Within a trauma-informed approach, amplifying the client's voice and providing meaningful choices encourages self-advocacy and reinforces the individual's sense of agency.

It's also essential to incorporate a strengths-based approach, recognizing and affirming the client's resilience, skills, and coping abilities. Appreciating what clients have overcome and the strengths they bring to the table can instill hope and a positive self-concept, which is key to healing from trauma.

Recognizing the widespread impact of trauma and understanding potential paths for recovery is another guiding light. As professionals, it's vital to appreciate the pervasiveness of trauma and its profound effects on individuals and communities. A broad perspective enables us to identify trauma responses and tailor interventions effectively.

Lastly, confronting issues related to secondary traumatic stress is important for practitioners. This means recognizing the emotional strain that can come from working with individuals who have experienced trauma, and taking steps to care for one's professional health as part of providing trauma-informed care.

When applied, these principles shift the clinical approach from one that asks, "What's wrong with you?" to "What's happened to you?" This subtle yet powerful reframing acknowledges the impact of life events on current functioning and paves the way for a more compassionate and effective therapeutic process.

Fostering resilience and recognizing signs of trauma are also inherent in a trauma-informed approach. Therapists should work to help clients identify and build upon their innate capacity to bounce back and adapt in the face of adversity. By doing so, they help instill a lens of strength, rather than one of pathology.

Interweaving the principle of collaboration involves the integration of family members, other healthcare providers, and community resources when appropriate. A multi-faceted network supports the client's healing and underscores the trauma-informed tenet of establishing connections.

The principles of a trauma-informed approach are interdependent and best practiced in synergy. They form a map that guides the therapeutic journey, ensuring that every step taken considers the intricate landscape of trauma and its aftermath.

As we envelop these principles into our practice, we commit to an ongoing process of learning, reflection, and adaptation. With these principles as our compass, we not only guide others toward healing but also affirm our dedication to a compassionate, conscious, and comprehensive practice that honors the complexities of the human spirit.

The Therapeutic Relationship and Safety

In the previous chapter, we unpacked the principles of a trauma-informed approach. As we continue our journey into the Foundations of Trauma-Informed Therapy, we must underscore the critical role of the therapeutic relationship and its bearing on safety. Crafting an environment where safety is not just an abstract concept but a tangible reality is central to any successful trauma-informed therapy.

The establishment of a therapeutic relationship begins with trust, and for individuals who have experienced trauma, trust can be elusive. A cornerstone of our role as therapists is to embody reliability, consistency, and respect. It's about gently inviting our clients into a space where they can start to believe that it's possible to engage with others without harm.

Imagine a sanctuary, a place where the travails and terrors of the past don't just recede; they are acknowledged and held with tender regard. This is what we work towards when we talk about safety within the therapeutic relationship. Safety is not merely the absence of threat but the presence of connection, understanding, and predictability.

For someone who has lived through trauma, the body and mind are often in a state of hypervigilance. As therapists, we must be acutely aware of our own presence—the words we choose, the tone of our voice, and our body language. Subtle cues that convey calm, non-judgment, and approachability can have a monumental impact on the felt sense of safety.

Engendering safety also involves boundaries—clear, compassionate, and consistently maintained. Boundaries are not just for our clients; they safeguard the therapeutic relationship and ensure that we, too, can operate from a place of steadiness and profession-alism. Transparent discussions about confidentiality, session structure, and professional limits all lay the groundwork for a secure alliance.

Within this sacred relationship, we adopt an attitude of curiosity rather than assumption. We listen with intent, seeking to understand the depths of the person before us. As we listen, we invite our clients to not only share their stories but also to recognize their own survival, strength, and agency. This strengths-based perspective is at the heart of empowerment, another key pillar in trauma-informed therapy.

Cultural humility also figures prominently in establishing safety. Recognizing and honoring diversity means understanding that our clients' experiences and perceptions are shaped by myriad social and cultural factors. It requires us to actively educate ourselves and to be open to learning from our clients about their unique contexts.

In this alliance, the term 'client-centered' takes on a profound significance. The goals, the pace, and the path of therapy are all determined in collaboration with the client. We're in this together, and every step forward is co-created. We're not just therapists; we're witnesses to the journey of healing and facilitators of change.

Our responses to our clients' narratives are pivotal. Offering validation without intrusion, empathizing without overwhelming—

these are the nuanced skills that help forge a bond that can endure the rigors of working through trauma. It is through this secure attachment that often develops in therapy that clients find a model for healthier relationships outside the therapeutic setting as well.

Safety in the therapeutic relationship also touches upon physical considerations. The therapy room itself must be a comforting and secure environment. The arrangement of chairs, the option of where to sit, the lighting and decor—these all contribute to a sense of safety and control for the client.

Educating our clients about the process of therapy and what they can expect is another way to establish safety. Demystification is empowering. When clients know that they can ask questions, express concerns, and provide feedback, they gain a voice in a process that might previously have felt opaque or intimidating to them.

We must also be attentive to triggers and work assiduously to avoid re-traumatization. As we get to know our clients, we become more adept at recognizing potential triggers and can plan our interventions with a careful eye toward safety. The practice of grounding techniques and coping strategies should be woven seamlessly into the fabric of therapy.

Self-regulation is essential for both therapist and client. As therapists, we must model self-regulation, engaging in practices that keep us grounded and centered, so that we can be present in a way that creates a regulating effect for our clients. In turn, we teach and empower our clients to discover and practice self-regulation strategies that work for them.

For healing to occur within the therapeutic relationship, there must also be a sense of hope—a belief that recovery is possible. Our optimism as therapists is not blind; it is fueled by the evidence of our clients' resilience and the transformation we are privileged to witness every day. This hope is contagious, and it becomes an integral part of the healing milieu we offer.

In sum, the therapeutic relationship is the bedrock foundation upon which trauma-informed therapy is built. It is within this relationship that safety is constructed, brick by brick, through trust, empathy, boundaries, curiosity, cultural humility, client-centered collaboration, and hope. As we continue to explore the layers of trauma-informed therapy, let's hold on to this truth: it is the quality of the therapeutic relationship that often determines the outcome of our efforts. As such, we must approach it with the reverence and dedication it deserves.

Creating an Environment of Empowerment

In the journey of trauma-informed therapy, the destination is not merely healing but empowerment. Trauma can strip away a person's sense of control and agency, making the restoration of these elements critical for recovery. Empowerment in a therapeutic context is the process of helping people to see their own strength, to make choices, and to influence their environment. It's not simply about obtaining power, but recognizing and cultivating the power within.

An environment of empowerment starts with the foundation of safety, which was discussed in the preceding section. Once safety is established, we focus on helping clients regain a sense of control over their lives, a process that is very much at the heart of trauma-informed therapy. In empowering our clients, we encourage them to rediscover their intrinsic motivation and foster autonomy—a stark contrast to the powerlessness that often characterizes traumatic experiences.

Empowerment is a collaborative endeavor. The therapeutic relationship should reflect a partnership where clients are not passive recipients, but active participants in their healing journey. This partnership requires us to engage with our clients with transparency, offering them choices and voicing our actions and intentions. Such clarity nurtures trust and reinforces the client's role in directing their own therapy.

Therapists should aim to highlight clients' strengths rather than solely focusing on pathology. By identifying and affirming the strengths that have helped clients survive their trauma, therapists foster resilience and promote a self-concept that encompasses both vulnerability and power. It is their resilience, after all, that has carried them to the point of seeking therapy.

Empowerment also involves skill building. Skills in emotion regulation, mindfulness, and interpersonal communication can all serve to elevate a sense of self-efficacy. As our clients learn and apply these skills, they begin to feel more capable of managing their symptoms and facing their trauma narrative.

Goal setting is another pivotal aspect of creating an environment of empowerment. We encourage clients to identify personal goals that are meaningful to them, helping them move beyond mere survival to thriving. Goals should be approached flexibly, reframing setbacks not as failures but as opportunities for learning and growth.

We must also recognize the socio-cultural factors that impact our clients' sense of empowerment. A trauma-informed therapist should understand and address issues such as access to resources, discrimination, and systemic barriers that might influence a client's ability to feel powerful. Efforts to empower the individual must be context-sensitive and culturally informed.

Consistent validation is a powerful tool in this process. Our clients need to feel seen and heard, and it's our role as therapists to provide that validation. Through empathetic listening and reflective responses, we affirm their experiences and feelings, further elevating their sense of self-worth.

In a similar vein, client feedback should be sought and valued. Their input on the therapeutic process not only fine-tunes the approach to suit their unique needs but also reaffirms their role as the expert in their own experiences. This shared decision-making model encapsulates the essence of empowerment.

Education is empowerment. Clients benefit from understanding trauma and its effects, the reasoning behind therapeutic interventions, and the expected trajectory of their recovery. An informed client is better equipped to actively participate in their treatment and make informed choices about their care.

The physical environment also plays a role in empowerment. Therapy spaces should be arranged to feel welcoming and respectful, fostering a sense of dignity. This also extends to scheduling and administrative practices—clients should find the logistical aspects of therapy accessible and accommodating.

Recognize that empowerment doesn't happen overnight. It is an evolving process that can be facilitated but not forced. Patience and perseverance are key as clients navigate this terrain at their own pace, and setbacks are a normal part of the journey towards reclaiming power.

It's important, too, to empower oneself as a therapist. Reflective practice ensures that we are aware of our own emotions and biases and how these may impact the therapy process. By doing so, we model self-empowerment—demonstrating to our clients that the quest for personal power and agency is a universal and lifelong pursuit.

Foster a network of support. While the therapist-client relationship is critical, drawing on community resources, support groups, and other networks can help to amplify the client's feelings of empowerment. This communal approach can bolster a client's self-efficacy and provide a multifaceted support system.

Lastly, celebrate progress, no matter how small. Recognizing and taking joy in the steps our clients take towards empowerment can serve as a powerful motivator for continued growth. It validates their efforts and strengths, reinforcing the ideal that they have the power to change their narrative.

The aim of creating an environment of empowerment is to set the stage for clients to emerge from the role of trauma survivors to that of architects of their own future. As facilitators of this transformative process, our role is to illuminate the path, provide the tools, and stand by as a testament to the power of the human spirit to overcome and flourish, despite adversity.

Chapter 3:
Assessment Strategies in Trauma Therapy

C ontinuing our journey into the heart of trauma therapy, we reach a pivotal stage where assessment not only informs but shapes the therapeutic path. A clinician's acuity in **assessing the symptoms and severity** of trauma directly impacts the effectiveness of the intervention. This phase calls for a specialized focus and sensitivity, akin to a cartographer charting unknown territories. Each survivor's experience is a unique terrain with its distinct topography of scars, and it's our role to map it out with precision, care, and an unyielding commitment to their healing. Truly effective assessment in trauma therapy isn't just clinical; it's an art that respects the individuality of each person's pain. In this chapter, we delve into the depths of **evaluating symptoms**, deploying **culturally sensitive assessment techniques**, and intricately weaving these threads into a **case conceptualization**. Here, the underpinning goal remains constant: to lay a bedrock of understanding so strong that it holds the weight of rebuilding lives. Through this delicate inquiry, we aim to discern the subtle nuances of each survivor's story, recognizing that a survivor's voice can only resonate in an environment built on trust, validation, and empathetic attunement. Let us then approach this task with an unwavering dedication to nuanced care, allowing us to illuminate the path toward hope and healing with every step of our collaborative exploration.

Evaluating the Symptoms and Severity

Assessment serves as the compass for the healing journey in trauma therapy. As mental health professionals, one of the most crucial skills to harness is the ability to evaluate symptoms and severity of a client's trauma. This assessment is a multi-faceted process requiring sensitivity, precision, and a clear understanding of the vast ways in which trauma can impact an individual.

The process begins with a thorough intake and evaluation. Clinicians must listen intently, not only to the words that are spoken but also to the subtleties that lie within the client's narrative. Remember, trauma imprints itself not just in the mind but also in the body, and often in ways that defy direct verbal articulation. By observing body language, emotional responses, and the ebb and flow of the client's storytelling, therapists can gather vital information about the depth and breadth of the traumatic impact.

Identifying the symptoms of trauma is to understand its diverse presentations. Some clients may exhibit clear post-traumatic stress disorder symptoms such as flashbacks, hyperarousal, and avoidance behaviors. Others may present with less specific symptoms like somatic complaints, generalized anxiety, or an inability to form secure attachments. It's important to approach each client with an open mind, acknowledging that trauma doesn't have a one-size-fits-all set of symptoms. Recognizing this variety is an integral part of establishing the severity of the trauma and the subsequent tailoring of treatment strategies.

Assessing the severity of trauma also involves looking at the client's functional impairment in their day-to-day life. Questionnaires and standardized scales may be employed, but they must be complemented by genuine human engagement. It's often through casual conversation that a client reveals the true extent to which traumatic symptoms have commandeered their ability to work, love, and play. These revelations can't be captured in a checkbox—they are found in the nuances of a shared human experience.

It is essential to conduct this assessment with an awareness of the individual's cultural and social context. Trauma does not exist in a vacuum. The individual's cultural background, gender identity, sexual orientation, and socioeconomic status all play significant roles in how they experience and articulate their trauma. This awareness is fundamental to an accurate and empathetic understanding of the client's lived experience and the unique ways in which trauma affects them.

Furthermore, a comprehensive assessment includes a historical perspective of the client's psychological, medical, and social history. Trauma can be insidious, often interwoven with past experiences and reinforced by subsequent events. A detailed history assists the therapist in discerning patterns, identifying triggers, and recognizing resilience and coping mechanisms that have either aided or impeded the client's natural capacity for healing.

Another aspect of evaluating symptoms and severity of trauma is acknowledging the potential for comorbid conditions. Trauma frequently coexists with other mental health disorders such as depression, substance abuse, and anxiety disorders. Careful differential diagnosis is vital to ensure that the treatment plan addresses all facets of the client's psychological health.

Client safety is paramount during the evaluation phase. Therapists must be vigilant regarding any signs of self-harm, suicidal ideation, or the potential for harm to others. Ensuring the individual is in a stable, safe condition to engage in therapy is a top priority before delving into the deeper work of trauma processing. If immediate safety concerns are present, these must be addressed with appropriate urgency and interventions.

Resilience factors such as social support, coping skills, and internal resources are equally significant when assessing the severity of trauma. These factors can be beacons of hope in a landscape often shadowed by pain and dysfunction. Recognizing and strengthening these resources is essential in building the therapeutic alliance and promoting healing.

Throughout the assessment, it's crucial to maintain transparency with the client. Let them know what you're observing, invite their input, and collaborate on the understanding of their symptoms. This shared assessment process fosters trust, empowers the client, and demystifies the therapeutic process. It also provides an opportunity to educate clients about the symptoms of trauma, which in itself can be therapeutic. Knowledge can transform the mysterious and terrifying symptoms into manageable and understandable reactions to past events, reducing the feeling of chaos and unpredictability.

Technology and its applications in assessment should not be overlooked. Whether it's through digital symptom tracking, online mental health platforms, or virtual reality tools, these modern technological aids can offer insights and metric data that complement traditional assessment methods.

As therapy progresses, remember that evaluating symptoms and severity is not a one-off task. It is an ongoing dialogue—a process that should be revisited at regular intervals in the therapeutic journey. Symptoms can evolve, and new layers of the trauma narrative may unearth additional complexities that require attention. Continuous assessment allows for treatment modalities to be adapted in real-time, ensuring that the approach remains relevant and effective.

Finally, embracing a strengths-based perspective when assessing trauma can be transformational. Encourage clients to recognize their resilience, commend them for their courage in seeking help, and reassure them that healing, though challenging, is within reach. This positive framing can fuel motivation and instill a sense of hope, both of which are invaluable on the path to recovery.

Assessing the symptoms and severity of trauma is both an art and a science. It requires a delicate balance of empathy, clinical expertise, cultural competence, and unwavering support. As therapists, we have the privilege and responsibility to hold space for our clients' pain while also casting light on their potential for healing and growth. The assessment is only the beginning, but it sets the foundation for the transformative work that lies ahead.

Culturally Sensitive Assessment Techniques

Understanding the rich tapestry of human experience is pivotal in trauma therapy. As professionals, we must be attuned to the cultural currents that shape the lives of those we serve. At the heart of this practice lies the imperative of culturally sensitive assessment - a complex yet rewarding endeavor.

Let's be clear: no single assessment method can encapsulate all cultural nuances. Instead, we must wield an array of techniques as gracefully as a painter wields their brush - with intention, knowledge, and genuine curiosity. Our goal is to sketch a portrait of the individual that honors their identity, experiences, and worldview.

Beginning with open-ended conversations, allow clients the space to share their personal narratives. It's through their stories that you'll gain insight into the cultural frameworks that hold meaning for them. As you listen, be aware of both what is said and what remains unspoken, as silence can carry as much weight as words.

In the context of trauma, remember that symptoms and their expressions can be heavily influenced by culture. What one community views as a normal reaction to distress, another might see as pathological. Therefore, it's imperative that we familiarize ourselves with various cultural interpretations of psychological symptoms.

Yet, it's not enough to simply recognize these differences - we must also respect them. Demonstrate your respect by asking clients about their comfort level with different aspects of the assessment process. Some may have reservations about particular approaches or questions, and it's our duty to adjust our methods accordingly.

Language represents a profound element of cultural identity. Where language barriers exist, ensure that interpreters are available, and be vigilant about the accuracy and subtlety of the interpretations. Miscommunication can not only compromise the assessment's efficacy but also the therapeutic relationship.

Consider also the role of nonverbal communication, which can be heavily influenced by culture. The meaning drawn from gestures, eye contact, and physical space can vary widely between cultural contexts. Cultivating an awareness of these variances allows for more nuanced interactions.

Beyond communication, explore the sociocultural factors that may contribute to trauma exposure and response. This entails an examination of societal structures, discrimination, historical oppression, and other contextual variables that might impact an individual's experience of trauma.

Use assessment tools that have been validated for use with diverse populations or, better yet, those specifically designed for the cultural group in question. This can help mitigate the risk of bias that often permeates tools developed within a single cultural framework.

However, we cannot entirely rely on these instruments. Practitioners must develop a critical eye, constantly evaluating the appropriateness of each tool. This entails a commitment to ongoing education and a willingness to consult with cultural informants or experts when needed.

Feedback is a gift, and in culturally sensitive assessments, it is invaluable. Engage clients in a discussion about the assessment process itself, seeking their perspective on what feels relevant, comfortable, and genuinely reflective of their experience.

Be aware of your own cultural lens and how it may color your interpretations. This requires a level of self-reflection and humility that's essential for growth as a trauma therapist. Engage in continuous self-assessment to monitor and manage your biases and assumptions.

Remember, building rapport is the cornerstone of effective assessment. It is forged through demonstrating empathy, expressing genuine interest in the client's cultural background, and providing validation. It's about creating an environment where clients truly feel seen and understood.

In the journey to cultivate cultural competence, it's important to acknowledge that it is a process, not a destination. We must be lifelong learners and remain adaptable in our approaches. It is through this dedication that we can provide assessments that not only inform but also affirm and empower.

At the crossroads of culture and trauma, there is an opportunity to serve as a catalyst for healing. As you refine your culturally sensitive assessment techniques, you forge a path toward a more inclusive, compassionate, and effective practice. Assess with care, and you'll undoubtedly make an indelible positive impact on the lives of those who brave your office seeking solace and strength.

Building a Case Conceptualization

Case conceptualization in trauma therapy is a pivotal step that provides a roadmap to understanding a client's unique experiences and symptoms, and to planning effective therapeutic interventions. It integrates information gathered during assessment and connects the theoretical understanding of trauma with the practice of therapy. Let's dive into the systematic approach to building a comprehensive case conceptualization for individuals who have endured trauma.

A starting point is the careful integration of a client's history and presenting concerns. As clinicians, we must listen deeply to the narratives shared, recognizing the patterns of thought, emotion, and behavior that reveal the impact of traumatic experiences. It's through empathetic attunement that we can truly understand the depth of the client's pain and start to envisage a path towards healing.

Next, an effective case conceptualization requires us to weave together the biological, psychological, and social threads that compose the fabric of the individual's life. Trauma often leaves a multi-dimensional mark, affecting clients on all these levels. Acknowledging the neurobiological effects of trauma, for instance, positions us to appreciate how trauma may manifest somatically, guiding relevant therapeutic interventions.

Critical to our conceptualization is identification of the types of trauma experienced—acute, chronic, or complex—and how these forms have interacted over time to shape the individual's current functioning. This nuanced understanding informs the tailoring of therapy to individual needs, ensuring that the approach is comprehensive and compassionate.

In building our case conceptualization, we cannot overlook the influence of culture, identity, and context. Culturally sensitive assessment techniques should have provided a foundation for recognizing how culture influences the experience and expression of trauma, as well as how it impacts a client's healing journey. This cultural attunement can inform a more informed and respectful therapeutic planning.

Relational dynamics represent another cornerstone of case conceptualization. A person's attachment history, including disruptions and their consequences, significantly informs their trauma response and relationships, including the therapeutic one. A thorough case conceptualization will reflect these dynamics and guide therapeutic endeavors to address and potentially heal attachment wounds.

When building the conceptualization, it's also important to consider comorbidities and how they interact with trauma symptoms. Often, clients present with additional disorders such as anxiety or depression, which intertwine with their trauma responses, necessitating a well-thought-out, integrated treatment approach.

Identifying strengths and resources is not merely an optimistic gesture; it is an integral part of the conceptualization process. Even in the depths of trauma, clients possess unique talents, relationships, and past successes that can be harnessed in the service of their recovery. Building on these strengths fosters resilience and empowers clients as active participants in their therapeutic journey.

A case conceptualization must be dynamic, updated regularly as more information comes to light or as the client progresses in therapy. Such flexibility ensures that the therapeutic approach remains relevant and responsive to the client's evolving needs, a testament to the personalized care inherent in trauma therapy.

We also integrate into conceptualization the knowledge of systemic and societal factors that impact the client, such as socioeconomic status or experiences of marginalization. This awareness allows us to situate the individual's experiences within a broader context, acknowledging external pressures and advocating for systemic change where necessary.

Treatment goals, derived from a clear case conceptualization, should be specific, measurable, achievable, relevant, and time-bound (SMART). These goals can give direction to the therapeutic process and a means to gauge progress, while also providing motivation and hope for clients. They let clients know that their healing journey has a destination, and that they're moving steadily towards it.

Another dimension of building case conceptualization includes considering potential treatment barriers and developing strategies to overcome them. These barriers could be internal, such as resistance or fear, or external, like a lack of support systems. Proactively addressing these barriers as part of the conceptualization can lead to more effective therapy.

Documentation in case conceptualization must be thorough, well-organized, and continuously updated. Detailed notes provide a reference point for both therapist and client, allowing for the tracking of therapeutic progress and ensuring that each session builds on the last.

Engaging clients in the construction of their case conceptualization can be empowering. By inviting their insights and perspectives, we promote a collaborative therapeutic relationship and honor their expertise on their lived experience. This shared journey fosters trust and cooperation, elements that are key to a transformative therapeutic process.

Lastly, building a case conceptualization isn't an academic exercise; it's a deeply human endeavor that serves as a beacon guiding the therapeutic journey. It should be a living document that reflects the continual interplay between theory and the tangible reality of each client's life. The ultimate aim is to provide a blueprint for healing, transformation, and wellbeing.

With these perspectives in mind, let us hold the case conceptualization as the heart of trauma therapy—a tool to understand, a framework to navigate, and a reflection of the unique story each client brings into our therapeutic space. As we embrace this crucial part of the healing journey, we walk alongside our clients with clarity and purpose, every step of the way.

Chapter 4:
Attachment Theory and Trauma

In the crucible of early development, the threads of attachment are delicately woven, forming the fabric of our future interactions and emotional landscape. Delving into the profound intersection of attachment theory and trauma, this chapter elucidates the pivotal role secure attachments play as both a bulwark against trauma and a cornerstone in the recovery process. It's in the understanding that disruptions in these early relationships can precipitate a vulnerability to trauma, altering one's ability to navigate stress and potentially contributing to lasting emotional turmoil. Yet, this is no path of despair; it's a journey towards enlightenment and healing. As mental health professionals, it's our privilege to guide clients toward reestablishing secure attachments through therapeutic methods, leading to a place where trust, safety, and resilience can flourish anew. This chapter strives to empower you with the wisdom to discern the nuances of attachment-oriented interventions and the tools to meticulously repair the intricate tapestry of the human connection when it has frayed under the weight of trauma.

The Role of Attachment in Trauma Response

In the landscape of trauma therapy, attachment theory has shifted from being just another lens through which to understand client experiences to a crucial framework for unpacking the complexities of trauma response. It brings forth a meaningful context that explains why some individuals, when faced with adversity, exhibit resilience while others succumb to the overwhelming forces of their experiences. The seminal works of John Bowlby and Mary Ainsworth on attachment offer much-needed bearings in this quest for delivering effective trauma-informed care.

Attachment—the emotional bond that develops between an infant and their primary caretaker—forms the blueprint for interpreting the world and self throughout one's life. Insecure attachments, whether they be avoidant, ambivalent, or disorganized, predispose individuals to a greater risk of difficulties when dealing with traumatic stressors. Their internalized views about self-worth and the reliability of others can dramatically skew their trauma responses.

A secure attachment cultivates a sense of safety, which is fundamental in navigating one's social world. When that is disrupted by trauma, the chosen strategies for coping can be profoundly affected. Those with secure attachments are generally more equipped to seek out support and confront their traumas in adaptive ways, engaging proactively in their healing journey.

Individuals who have suffered from chronic or complex trauma, particularly in early life, often endure significant disruptions in their attachment patterns. Perhaps they've encountered inconsistent responses from caregivers, or their cries for help have been systematically ignored or met with hostility. As therapists, it is our task not just to recognize these patterns but to appreciate the weighty implications they carry for the therapeutic process.

In considering trauma response through the lens of attachment, we must see that a person's history is not merely a catalogue of events but is composed of relationships that have either fortified or eroded their foundation for resilience. Those who have not had the luxury of secure attachments may manage their distress using methods that, to the external world, appear maladaptive. However, within the frame of their lived experience, these methods provided necessary, if not vital, strategies for psychological survival.

Traumatic events can challenge or shatter one's attachment system, leading to feelings of disconnection, abandonment, and mistrust in relationships. For some, this involves the activation of older, less functional attachment strategies—like clinging, avoidance, or shutting down emotionally—as a reflexive guard against further pain. This emergent distress in attaching can culminate in profound difficulties, spanning from interpersonal relationships to one's capacity for emotional regulation.

Our therapeutic interventions should, therefore, be geared toward helping clients explore and understand their unique attachment histories. This allows us to tailor our approach to meet them where they are, providing the necessary support for them to grapple with their past traumas from a more anchored position. Healing within this domain fosters not only individual well-being but also enriches their relational worlds.

With the understanding that our clients' attachment systems have been taxed, if not torn, by their traumatic experiences, our therapeutic presence can be the reparative base from which they can start to rebuild. We become a transitional attachment figure, one that offers consistency, attunement, and responsive care, thus forging a pathway towards the development of a secure attachment capacity within them.

For instance, we may utilize the therapeutic space to model what secure attachment looks like through our dependability, attunement to the client's needs and emotional states, and nonjudgmental acceptance. This form of corrective relational experience can be deeply healing, as it allows clients to develop trust in others and themselves, often for the first time. Notably, it is through these new relational experiences that clients can start to rewrite their internal working models of relationships.

Attachment theory also informs us about the potential transference and countertransference reactions that both clients and therapists may experience. As therapists, being cognizant of our attachment styles is just as imperative as understanding those of our clients. Our own patterns can unconsciously influence the therapeutic relationship and process, either facilitating growth or inadvertently perpetuating attachment insecurities.

Furthermore, the attachment lens reminds us that therapeutic change is not solely a cognitive enterprise. The relational aspect of therapy—being felt, heard, and understood—can attune clients to inner states that may have been dismissed or unacknowledged due to maladaptive attachment patterns. The therapeutic relationship becomes a vessel for embodying new ways of relating, thus contributing to a client's ability to modulate emotions and experiences more adaptively.

The work we engage in with clients who have experienced trauma is not just a matter of implementing treatment protocols; it is about being a steady compass in their storm, an anchor amidst tumultuous seas. The journey they embark on in therapy, guided by the principles of attachment theory, is one that has the potential to liberate them from the chains of their past, to transform their present, and courageously forge a future replete with connections that are secure, enriching, and supportive.

Ultimately, as therapists, we are uniquely positioned to influence the quality of our clients' relational matrices, which, in turn, shapes their ability to cope with stress and trauma. This work is profound. It requires our utmost presence, empathetic attunement, and endless reservoirs of compassion. By integrating attachment theory into our trauma-informed practices, we touch the very core of what it means to be human—the innate desire for secure connections, understanding, and growth.

At the kernel of trauma and attachment theory is hope—the notion that bonds can be mended, that security can emerge from chaos, and that our clients can and will find their way back to their authentic selves, fortified by the knowledge that they are worthy of love and capable of forging lasting, healing connections.

Addressing Attachment Disruptions

Our understanding of trauma's profound impact brings us squarely to the heart of attachment theory. When disrupted by traumatic experiences, the attachment systems that govern our relationships and sense of security in the world can become disorganized or insecure. As therapists, we are in a unique position to engage with these deep-seated attachment wounds and foster an environment where healing can begin to take root.

Attachment disruption can be likened to the uprooting of a tree, which once stood firmly integrated within its environment. Trauma, much like a violent storm, can disturb the rootedness of this tree, causing instability and disconnection. In humans, this manifests as difficulty in maintaining relationships, distrust, anxiety, or an inability to self-regulate emotions effectively.

One of the first steps in addressing attachment disruptions is recognizing the signs in our clients. The subtleties in their interactions, narratives of past relationships, and current relational patterns provide windows into their attachment styles. Are they avoidant, dismissing closeness and connection? Perhaps they are anxious, seeking constant validation and clinging to relationships out of fear? Or are they disorganized, displaying a confusing mix of behaviors indicative of mixed and unresolved feelings towards attachment figures?

Approaching these clients requires patience and empathy. The therapeutic relationship itself becomes a crucible for change, where trust must be painstakingly built and the fear of closeness must be gently challenged. As therapists, we hold the space for clients to explore their vulnerabilities without judgment, modeling the secure base they may have lacked.

Our work then turns to helping our clients understand their own attachment patterns. Making these unconscious patterns conscious empowers individuals to see how their past is influencing their present. Through our therapeutic alliance, we can provide corrective emotional experiences, those small but critical moments where clients feel understood, supported, and valued in new and profound ways.

Psychoeducation plays a critical role in the healing process. Helping clients learn about their attachment style can bring tremendous relief. They're not flawed or irreparably broken; they've adapted to their past environments in the best way they knew how. With this knowledge, clients can begin to see a path forward, one that involves creating new experiences and expectations around relationships.

As we delve deeper into attachment work, we turn our attention to the body. Trauma is stored somatically, and attachment disruptions often manifest through physiological responses. Assisting clients in developing a mindful awareness of their bodies provides them with an invaluable tool in managing and understanding their emotional reactions.

Attachment-focused therapy often involves revisiting past traumas. This work must be done with care, ensuring clients have developed sufficient coping strategies to manage the distress that may arise. Through carefully paced exposure and processing of past events, we are helping clients to reframe their experiences and understand them in the context of their attachment needs.

Healing from attachment disruptions also necessitates the development of self-compassion. Clients may carry deep-seated beliefs about their unworthiness or unlovability stemming from early attachment traumas. Encouraging self-love is vital, as is the process of re-parenting oneself by providing the care and nurture that was missing.

It's important to recognize that attachment healing does not occur in isolation. Encouraging clients to build secure connections outside of therapy is also part of the therapeutic journey. We promote the gradual building of relationships that are safe and affirming, whether through reconnecting with trustworthy family members, cultivating friendships, or engaging in community activities.

The path of healing from attachment disruptions is incremental and challenging, yet deeply rewarding. As clients start to internalize new ways of relating and experiencing the world, we witness moments of triumph. A once and pervasive sense of isolation gives way to a blossoming belief in the possibility of connection and the experience of joy in relationships.

Throughout this healing process, we must brace ourselves with patience, reminding clients that setbacks are part of the journey. The ruptures that inevitably occur offer precious opportunities for repair, further solidifying the client's learning and growth in attachment security.

We must also attend to cultural and individual differences in attachment and trauma. A one-size-fits-all approach has no place in trauma therapy. Each client brings a unique narrative shaped by their cultural background, family dynamics, and personal experiences. As therapists, we must honor and integrate these differences into our approach to attachment repair.

Finally, the progress in attachment healing, at times, seems to emerge not in grand, sweeping changes, but in the subtle shifts in a client's way of being. A softened gaze, the courage to ask for help, or a moment of genuine laughter shared with another; these are the markers of healing that, when accumulated, represent a reorientation of one's attachment world.

The journey of reparation and growth within attachment disruptions is an arduous one, but it is also a testament to the resilience and adaptability of the human spirit. As therapists, our role is to guide, support, and bear witness to the incredible capacity individuals possess to reconcile with their past and to build a foundation for healthier, more secure attachments in their future.

Therapeutic Approaches to Rebuild Secure Attachments

In the realm of trauma therapy, restoring secure attachments stands as a cornerstone of the healing process. For an individual who has experienced traumatic disruption in early attachments, the therapeutic relationship itself can serve as a reparative experience. Echoing the safe haven that was once compromised, this section will illuminate the pathways through which we can foster secure attachments and catalyze deep, lasting healing.

The bedrock of rebuilding secure attachments lies in the consistency and reliability of the therapeutic setting. Therapists can create a sense of safety by being predictably available and responsive, mirroring the ideal attachment figure. This in itself can be profoundly restorative, as clients begin to internalize the experience of safety and develop a secure base within the therapy relationship.

Therapists often employ a technique known as "earned secure attachment." By engaging clients in a corrective emotional experience, therapists replace their expectations of fear and abandonment with anticipations of support and attunement. Establishing an earned secure attachment demands patience, as the therapist gently guides the client back from the relational edges where trauma resides.

Another fundamental approach involves identifying and exploring patterns of attachment behavior in therapy. Clients may project onto the therapist patterns formed in early life, and by making these dynamics explicit, both therapist and client can work together to understand and transform them. It's not just about recognizing patterns, but fostering new ways of relating that encourage trust, collaboration, and mutual respect.

Mindfulness and present-moment awareness can significantly enhance the therapeutic bond and help clients tune into their own emotional states. By focusing on here-and-now experiences, clients learn to observe their reactions to attachment-related distress without judgment. This mindfulness strategy empowers individuals to pause and choose more adaptive responses in their relationships.

Therapists can also integrate attachment narratives in the healing journey. Engaging clients in storytelling about their past attachment experiences allows them to reconstruct their understanding of relationships and self. Cognitive narrative techniques such as coherence therapy help clients weave together fragmented memories into a more cohesive and empowering life story.

Sensorimotor psychotherapy introduces body awareness as a tool to strengthen the therapeutic attachment. Through gentle body-centered interventions, clients can develop an embodied sense of safety and connectedness. This somatic avenue can often reach layers of attachment trauma that purely cognitive approaches may miss.

Rebuilding secure attachments isn't exclusively an intrapsychic journey; it also involves real-world relationship practice. Therapists may encourage clients to engage in new relational experiences outside of therapy that serve to reinforce a sense of security in interactions with others. Gradually, through this "relational rehearsal," individuals transfer their secure base from the therapy room to their wider social world.

The therapeutic concept of "mentalization" is particularly impactful in attachment-focused therapy. By fostering mentalizing abilities, therapists help clients to better understand their own and others' mental states. This reflective function is integral to forming secure attachments and navigating interpersonal dynamics effectively.

For those whose attachment trauma relates to familial bonds, family therapy modalities can be pivotal. Techniques such as family systems therapy offer a platform for resolving conflicts and building healthier interaction patterns. These interventions can powerfully shift familial attachments towards greater security and resilience.

Attachment-informed EMDR (Eye Movement Desensitization and Reprocessing) is rapidly becoming an asset in the trauma therapist's toolkit. Incorporating attachment theory into EMDR's structured approach renders it uniquely effective in processing trauma and fostering secure attachment simultaneously. Clients can thus reprocess distressing memories while being supported by the robust therapeutic alliance formed.

Psychoeducation also plays a valuable role in reconstructing secure attachments. By understanding the principles of attachment theory, clients gain insights into their relationship styles and challenges. Knowledge is empowering, and when clients comprehend the 'why' behind their feelings and behaviors, they can engage more meaningfully in the process of change.

Therapists may also draw upon experiential therapies, such as psychodrama or Gestalt techniques, to give clients a live platform to explore and repair attachment wounds. By acting out past situations or adopting roles that were absent or distorted in their own lives, clients can confront unresolved emotions and initiate corrective healing experiences.

A collaborative approach ties all these methods together, with the therapist and client working as a team. It's essential that clients feel they have a voice and choice in their therapy. Mutual goal setting, empowerment, and a shared commitment to healing strengthen the therapeutic attachment and reinforce the client's autonomy and capability.

Ultimately, as therapists, we are sculptors of hope. Our role is to help clients shape their internal worlds from one of chaos and fear to one of congruence and security. By thoughtfully integrating attachment-focused interventions, we provide the supportive scaffolding that enables individuals to build robust, secure attachments and manifest a resilient, fulfilling life beyond the shadows of their trauma.

Chapter 5:
Somatic Approaches to Trauma Resolution

As we delve deeper into the therapeutic odyssey of trauma healing, we arrive at the phenomenally potent domain of *Somatic Approaches to Trauma Resolution*. In this chapter, we journey through the landscape of the body, exploring its silent narratives and unlocking the wisdom enshrined within our very sinews and cells. Therapists like you stand at the vanguard, guiding those who have been shackled by their past traumas towards liberation through the transformative power of somatic practices. Concepts such as somatic experiencing invite an intimate dialogue between mind, body, and emotion, ushering in profound healing. Acknowledge the body as a vessel that has held and sometimes hidden deep-seated anguish, and equip yourself with techniques that gently coax it to release these burdens. As practitioners, we wield the artful balance of science and intuition to reacquaint individuals with their bodies' inherent capacity to recuperate and flourish, championing a holistic renaissance that honors the indomitable spirit of human resilience. Your gentle, attuned guidance can light the path to renewal, inviting each breath, each movement to contribute to the grand tapestry of recovery. Therein, the body becomes a gateway to emancipation from trauma's oppressive grip, promising a return to vitality and a reclamation of serenity. Embrace this chapter as an in-depth exploration of how the somatic realm can be both a crucible for trauma and a sanctuary for healing.

The Body's Narratives: Somatic Memory

As we delve into the realm of somatic experiencing, we acknowledge the profound narratives that our bodies carry – narratives rich with the wisdom of lived experience and often the weight of trauma. These somatic memories, encoded within our very tissues, present a language beyond words. They narrate stories of our past encounters, battles fought, and wounds sustained, giving shape to how we interact with the world at large.

Somatic memory refers to the physiological imprint of emotional and traumatic events, which, despite passing time, remain etched into our bodies. Unlike explicit memory, which includes conscious recollections of facts or events, somatic memories consist of sensations, impulses, and motor patterns that can be triggered even without a conscious correlation to the original trauma.

Consider, for instance, how a particular scent can transport someone back to a childhood kitchen or how an unexpected touch may evoke a sense of danger based on past experiences. These are the silent whispers of somatic memory, communicating in the currency of bodily responses.

For many of our clients, these memories are not only dormant heirlooms of their history but active participants in their daily lives. They contribute to their reactivity, preferences, and often inexplicable aversions. The task at hand for clinicians is to aid clients in deciphering these visceral messages, to tenderly unlock the tight script of body memories, and ultimately assist in rewriting their embodied narrative toward healing.

One way to access somatic memory is through techniques that gently probe the body's story. Practices like mindful body scanning, where individuals attune to the sensations within their bodies, can reveal tensions and patterns associated with unprocessed traumas.

These bodily cues are portals into the internal world that might otherwise remain unexamined.

In attending to somatic memory, we must also honor the body's innate intelligence and its capacity for self-regulation and healing. The body often knows what is needed before the mind has a chance to articulate it, and as therapists, fostering a deep respect and curiosity for the body's communications forms the cornerstone of somatic therapy.

It's essential that clinicians themselves maintain a grounded, present, and embodied state. Doing so acts as a mirror for clients, offering them a relational home base from which they can learn to navigate their own internal physiological stirrings with greater ease and awareness. This form of modeling is imperative, as it demonstrates the power of being in one's body rather than dissociating from it.

A key part of somatic approaches involves helping clients develop awareness of how their bodies respond to stress and calming cues. This psychoeducation about the body's physiological responses equips individuals with knowledge that can be empowering – transforming feelings of helplessness into a sense of agency over one's own body and, by extension, one's emotional state.

Therapeutic interventions targeting somatic memory may include breathwork, movement therapies, or somatic experiencing techniques that help to discharge and integrate these memories. Clients learn to oscillate between resources and discomfort, navigating their history not as a behemoth to be slain but as a terrain to be understood and traversed with compassion.

In working with somatic memories, grounding techniques become pivotal. By anchoring individuals in the present moment, we help them differentiate past experiences from current realities. Simple acts like feeling one's feet on the ground or touching a textured object can serve as powerful anchors, reassuring the nervous system that here and now is safe, even if the past was fraught with danger.

Alongside grounding, titration is a key concept in processing somatic memories. Rather than diving into traumatic experiences all at once – which can be re-traumatizing – titration allows for a gradual approach. This process respects the client's pace, building tolerance to distressing emotions and sensations in doses that can be metabolically processed.

As practitioners, our role is to create a therapy space that feels affirming and nurturing, where somatic memories can surface, be felt, and expressed without fear of judgment. In this space, clients can experiment with new postures and movements that challenge old patterns and begin to codify new experiences in their bodies.

When therapists guide clients through the mazes of their somatic narratives, they guide them towards transformation. Somatic memory work is not just about revisiting the past; it's also about embodying a more integrated and harmonious future. This is where the paths of resilience and embodiment intersect, where clients start to inhabit their bodies with empowerment rather than trepidation or pain.

The pathway of healing through somatic memory is a journey back to oneself. It's a reclaiming of the body as a sanctuary after it has felt like a battleground. Healing asks for patience, presence, and often, the courage to meet parts of oneself that have been long estranged. The beauty of this journey is not only in the destination but in the transformation that occurs step by reverent step.

In our work, we strive not only to unpack and understand the stories held within the bodies of those who seek our guidance but also to honor and bear witness to the incredible journey each individual embarks upon in the quest for wholeness. By helping clients re-narrate their somatic memories, we assist them in reclaiming their bodily autonomy, their inner strength, and their inherent capacity for healing.

Techniques in Somatic Experiencing

As we plunge deeper into the nuances of somatic approaches to trauma resolution, we must focus on specific techniques within Somatic Experiencing (SE). This powerful modality, developed by Dr. Peter Levine, acknowledges the profound connection between the body and the traumas it harbors. Through SE, practitioners are equipped with the methods necessary to facilitate the release of traumatic shock and the restoration of inner balance.

At the outset of employing Somatic Experiencing techniques, practitioners cultivate an environment of presence. It's essential for the therapist to be fully attentive, grounded, and attuned to the subtle cues of the client's body language, affect, and verbal communication. This presence helps to create a therapeutic space in which clients can begin to explore their trauma with safety and support.

One foundational aspect of SE is the concept of 'titration.' Much like a chemist who carefully measures out reagents to avoid an overwhelming reaction, the SE therapist introduces small amounts of traumatic material for the client to process. This prevents re-traumatization and ensures that the client is not flooded with intense emotional responses all at once.

Pendulation, another key technique, refers to the gentle oscillation between states of activation and deactivation within the client's nervous system. As clients are guided to notice their sensations and reactions, they also learn to recognize their own capacities for self-regulation and resilience. The therapist's role here is akin to a compassionate guide, leading clients through the ebb and flow of their emotions and bodily sensations.

'Resourcing' is a term used in SE to signify the process of identifying and reinforcing elements within the client or their environment that provide comfort, strength, or a sense of stability. These resources can be anything from positive memories and personal strengths, to grounding exercises that foster a sense of safety and regulation.

Another technique, 'Completion of Fight-Flight Responses,' reengages the thwarted physical actions that were not possible during the initial traumatic event. This facilitates the release of pent-up survival energy and can often lead to a profound sense of relief for the client.

Building up 'Somatic Awareness' is crucial in SE. Clients are taught to attentively observe their bodily sensations, learning to decode the language of the body which often holds the keys to unresolved trauma. As clients enhance their somatic awareness, they can begin to discern between past and present, reducing the impact of traumatic memories.

SE therapy also utilizes what is called 'tracking.' This involves the therapist helping clients become aware of their moment-to-moment sensory experiences, anchoring them in the present and countering the disassociation that can accompany trauma. Through tracking, the narrative of trauma is steadily disentangled from the body's somatic responses.

'Containment and Grounding' techniques are practiced to foster a sense of security and stability within the client. Here, the client may be supported in creating imagined or physical boundaries, reinforcing the knowledge that they are in a safe space. Grounding techniques, such as deep breathing and mindful body scans, are key to maintaining this sense of containment.

SE doesn't overlook the power of the therapeutic relationship, and the technique of 'Co-regulation' leverages the connection between client and therapist. Through the therapist's calm and centered demeanor, clients can experience a model for nervous system regulation, enhancing their capacity for self-regulation over time.

In situations where trauma has resulted in a sense of loss or disconnection, Somatic Experiencing employs a technique known as 'Renegotiation.' Rather than simply revisiting the trauma, the client is guided toward new outcomes and empowered to envision alternative scenarios in which they experience agency and choice.

An important technique in SE is 'Discharge,' where clients are assisted in releasing stored energy in the body that relates to the trauma. This may manifest in the form of shaking, crying, or other forms of physical release, allowing the client to move through and beyond the 'stuck' energy.

'Integration' is the process that weaves together the new insights and equilibrium achieved through the various SE techniques. Integration ensures the stability of these changes and supports the gradual expansion of the client's capacity to engage with life's challenges without being overwhelmed by past trauma.

Lastly, 'Expansion,' a technique focused on capturing moments of relief or positive sensation in the body, steadily builds a foundation for a more enlivened and dynamic experience. Clients learn to savour these moments, which can gradually redefine their sense of self and their perception of the world as a safer place.

These SE techniques are not just isolated strategies but are interwoven into an empathic, attuned, and flexible approach to trauma therapy. As practitioners, we wield these techniques with the intent of not just healing trauma but also fostering a profound transformation in our clients' lives, encouraging them to reclaim their vitality and engage fully with the world around them.

Integrating Body Work into Trauma Therapy

The journey toward healing from trauma is a deeply personal and often complex path, where therapists have the profound responsibility of guiding their clients through the murky waters of past suffering. Recognizing that trauma lives not just in the mind but is also inscribed upon the body is a pivotal shift in the treatment of trauma. Integrating body work into trauma therapy can serve as a powerful catalyst in the process, helping to release the somatic echoes of traumatic events.

Understanding the body's role in trauma response is crucial. When someone experiences trauma, their sympathetic nervous system is activated, and they may become locked in a 'fight or flight' state. For some, this physiological arousal doesn't fully subside, even long after the threat is gone, leaving them with heightened stress responses that are somatically stored. This stored trauma can manifest in myriad ways, including chronic pain, tension, and other physical symptoms.

The integration of body work into trauma therapy begins with education. Therapists can help clients understand the somatic aspect of their trauma, nurturing an awareness that their physical symptoms are not simply manifestations of stress but are also deeply entwined with their emotional pain. This acknowledgment is empowering and an essential first step towards somatic healing.

Trauma-informed body work employs a variety of techniques to help release tension and restore regulation in the body's systems. These techniques might include somatic experiencing, mindful movement, and breathwork, among others. As a therapist, it's critical to collaborate with clients, allowing them to lead the way and set the pace, fostering a sense of safety and control that trauma often strips away.

Breathwork can serve as a gentle entry point to body work. Controlled breathing exercises can help regulate the autonomic nervous system, turning down the volume on hyperarousal and offering clients a direct way to influence their physiological state. Therapists should guide clients with empathy, recognizing that even the simplest breathwork can be intense for those with significant trauma.

Mindful movement, like yoga or tai chi, can also be integrated into therapy sessions. These practices help clients to reconnect with their bodies, often disowned and ignored in the aftermath of trauma. The slow deliberate movements are not just physical exercises, but opportunities for clients to experience their bodies without fear or discomfort.

Somatic Experiencing is another profound tool, developed by Peter Levine, to help release the 'stuck' energy and emotions from the body. It's a gentle process that involves noticing bodily sensations associated with trauma and then gradually helping the client to 'complete' the self-protective responses that were thwarted during the traumatic event.

Adding body work into therapy must be done with the utmost sensitivity to the individual's boundaries and comfort level. For some, touch-based therapies like massage or craniosacral therapy might be beneficial, but this requires a respectful and continuous checking-in with the client's comfort with physical contact. The therapist's primary role is to cultivate a space that feels secure for exploration and expression of somatic experiences.

Grounding techniques are integral to body work. These techniques help clients to manage dissociation and overwhelming emotions by reconnecting with the present moment. Grounding can include anything from feeling the weight of one's body in a chair to focusing on the sensation of feet pressing into the floor.

As therapists navigate this integration, they must hold space for emotional releases that often accompany somatic work. Tears, trembling, warmth, and an array of other physical reactions may surface as the body releases its grip on trauma, and these signs should be welcomed as part of the healing process.

Interoceptive awareness, or the ability to sense the internal state of the body, is a key skill that therapists can help clients develop. This awareness promotes a deeper connection with oneself and serves as an anchoring point in therapy. As clients become more attuned to their body's cues, they gain valuable insight into their emotional world.

Therapists must also be prepared to adjust their approach in response to client feedback. Integrating body work is a dynamic process that requires flexibility, patience, and attentiveness to the shifting comfort levels and needs of the client. It is a process of constant learning and adaptation.

It's paramount for therapists to work in tandem with other professionals who specialize in body-centered therapies when needed. A multidisciplinary team approach can maximize the benefits of somatic work and ensure that clients receive the specialized care they may need.

Lastly, but perhaps most importantly, the therapist's role is to empower clients in recognizing their own strength and resilience. Trauma therapy focused on body work emphasizes the remarkable capacity of the body to recover and restore. It is a profound journey that can reawaken hope and foster a renewed sense of freedom in one's physical and emotional existence.

Throughout this practice, it's vital to remain anchored in the principles of trauma-informed care, understanding that the journey is as unique as the individual embarking on it. Integrating body work into trauma therapy can be transformative, shedding the layers of pain held within the body and illuminating the path towards a healthier, more integrated self.

Chapter 6:
Cognitive and Behavioral Interventions

Delving into the landscape of cognitive and behavioral interventions, this sixth chapter illuminates the transformative pathways that empower those healing from trauma. As practitioners, we weave the fabric of resilience using threads of evidence-based practices like Cognitive Processing Therapy (CPT) and Dialectical Behavior Therapy (DBT) that are tailored to reframe and rebuild the ruptured schemas of traumatized individuals. The rich tapestry of therapeutic techniques continues with the exposure therapies, Prolonged Exposure (PE), and Eye Movement Desensitization and Reprocessing (EMDR) that navigate the labyrinth of traumatic memories, guiding clients towards the reclamation of their autonomous selves. Here, we shall explore the art and science of these interventions to not only alleviate the symptoms of trauma but also foster a renewed sense of mastery and hope in the lives touched by the echoes of their past.

Cognitive Processing Therapy (CPT)

As we delve into the specifics of cognitive and behavioral interventions in the treatment of trauma, we inevitably come across Cognitive Processing Therapy (CPT), a distinctive and evidence-based approach that has shown marked success in mitigating the symptoms of post-traumatic stress disorder (PTSD). Developed by Drs. Patricia Resick, Candice Monson, and Kathleen Chard, CPT embodies the notion that traumatic events challenge an individual's pre-existing beliefs about the world, themselves, and others, often leading to cognitive distortions that perpetuate the symptoms of PTSD.

Central to CPT is acknowledging that while traumatic events are not preventable by the individual who experienced them, the ongoing suffering is connected to the interpretations or stuck points that those individuals have about the event. By broadening the narrative of the trauma and examining these stuck points critically, CPT empowers individuals to reframe and reassess their thoughts and emotions surrounding their traumatic experience.

Consisting of 12 to 16 sessions, typically one hour each, CPT is conducted either individually or in group settings. The structured nature of CPT encapsulates a teaching component where clients first learn about the symptoms of PTSD and the relationship between thoughts and emotions, setting a foundation for the therapeutic work to come.

One of the acclaimed features of CPT is the introduction of the concept of 'Challenging Questions'. These questions serve as tools for individuals to interrogate and dissect the veracity of their beliefs about the traumatic event. Commonly, these maladaptive beliefs pertain to themes of safety, trust, power, control, esteem, and intimacy. By challenging these beliefs, clients begin to untangle the mental knots that the trauma has tied around their cognitive processes.

The process of writing is crucial in CPT. Patients are tasked with writing detailed accounts of their traumatic events, which serves two critical purposes: externalization of the trauma narrative and an opportunity for therapists to pinpoint key areas that need cognitive restructuring. As clients read these narratives aloud, it often diminishes the power of the traumatic memories, making them less overwhelming and more manageable.

Another key element is the identification and examination of 'automatic thoughts' – those immediate, knee-jerk reactions to external stimuli or internal emotions connected to the trauma. For example, a survivor of an assault may automatically think, "I am powerless," whenever they encounter situations that evoke vulnerability. CPT works to map out these automatic thoughts and teaches clients how to confront and modify them.

Throughout the therapy, clients actively engage in Socratic dialogue with their therapist – a dynamic exchange that fosters deep cognitive exploration and reframing. This dialogue is not simply a conversation; it is a technique through which therapists guide clients toward self-discovery and the reorganization of their traumatic beliefs.

It's fundamental in CPT to address feelings of guilt and self-blame. These feelings are common among people who have experienced trauma, and they can create profound barriers to recovery if left unchallenged. Through CPT, individuals can differentiate between guilt and responsibility, often leading to significant breakthroughs in treatment.

We must bear in mind that trauma disturbs the narrative of one's life, and CPT is about rewriting that narrative in a more balanced and realistic manner. It takes courage to revisit traumatic memories, but in doing so through CPT, clients are not only recounting what has happened, they are actively processing and transforming their story.

The homework assignments in CPT are not just supplemental; they're integral to the therapy's success. Assignments might include practice of the skills learned in sessions, daily thought records to capture and challenge problematic thinking, and the continuation of writing about the traumatic event. It nurtures the growth that happens outside the therapy room and encourages autonomy in the recovery process.

Research on CPT indicates significant reductions in PTSD symptoms for a variety of populations, including military veterans, sexual assault survivors, and individuals who have experienced complex trauma. Such outcomes illuminate the potent capability of this modality to not just treat PTSD, but also to enable individuals to understand and grow beyond their experiences.

Adaptability is also a noteworthy aspect of CPT. While it adheres to a structured protocol, there's room for tailoring the therapy to the unique cultural and individual needs of clients. Understanding that the lens through which we see the world is distinctively shaped by our background, CPT therapists are trained to navigate these nuances with sensitivity and respect.

Despite its many strengths, CPT is not a panacea and is not suitable for everyone. Therapists must use discernment to determine whether this modality is the best fit for a client, based on factors such as the individual's stability, readiness to process trauma narratives, and existing coping skills. Diligent assessment before commencement of therapy is vital to safeguard the best interests of the client.

Ultimately, the goal of CPT is not merely symptom reduction but fostering post-traumatic growth – the profound and overarching change that can occur following the struggle with traumatic events. This growth speaks to resilience, the ability to find meaning, and the development of richer life perspectives. CPT thus becomes a journey where individuals not only regain control over their lives but also discover strengths and insights that were previously veiled by the shadow of trauma.

In conclusion, Cognitive Processing Therapy caters to the deep-rooted cognitive distortions that often govern the lives of those suffering in the aftermath of trauma. As facilitators of healing, we strive to shine light on these shadows, so that those we serve may find their way back to a life of balance and hope. A practitioner's attunement to the delicate intricacies of their client's cognitive landscapes allows them to guide their journey through CPT with empathy, finesse, and an unwavering belief in their capacity for renewal.

Dialectical Behavior Therapy (DBT) for Trauma

In the realm of treatment for individuals who have faced trauma, Dialectical Behavior Therapy (DBT) emerges as a shining beacon, offering skills and strategies to enhance emotional and cognitive regulation. This chapter delves into the application of DBT in the context of trauma, weaving through its core components and illustrious techniques which pivot on the fulcrum of dialectical thinking—the reconciliation of opposites—to foster resilience and healing.

Originally conceived to treat Borderline Personality Disorder, DBT's profound impact has transcended its initial scope, revealing its versatility in addressing traumatic stress disorders. This speaks to the transformative power of DBT to adapt to the labyrinthine intricacies of the human psyche affected by trauma. It's a reminder that in the shadows of adversity, there is a path forward shaped by compassion, skillfulness, and an unwavering commitment to growth.

At the heart of DBT is the principle of dialectics, or the integration of opposites. The therapeutic process recognizes the client's need for acceptance of their experiences while simultaneously working towards change. This balancing act is delicate; it's about nurturing a sense of self-compassion in clients while challenging them to confront painful truths and develop new coping mechanisms.

DBT is anchored by four skill modules: mindfulness, distress tolerance, emotion regulation, and interpersonal effectiveness. Mindfulness practices in DBT serve as the backbone, enabling clients to remain present with their experiences, which is especially critical when traumatic memories and associated emotions threaten to overwhelm. With mindfulness, an inner sanctuary is cultivated—one where the storms of the past may be observed without yielding to their power to upset the equilibrium of the present.

The distress tolerance component offers a lifeline in moments where emotional turmoil runs high. It equips clients with practical tools to endure and survive crisis situations without resorting to harmful behaviors. It is about finding an oasis of calm within chaos, thus empowering clients to navigate their tempestuous internal seas with grace.

Emotion regulation skills in DBT provide the roadmap for understanding and managing intense emotions that trauma so often ignites. By learning to identify and label emotions accurately, clients gain leverage over impulsive reactions. They're taught to reshape their emotional responses to align with their aspirations for healing, fostering an emotional alchemy that transmutes pain into purposeful action.

Interpersonal effectiveness strategies broaden the therapeutic impact by focusing on navigating relationships. These skills are critical, as trauma can profoundly disrupt one's ability to trust and connect with others. By forging stronger communication abilities and assertiveness, clients can reconstruct healthy boundaries and engage more meaningfully with the world around them.

DBT embraces the enigmatic art of validation—recognizing and affirming the client's feelings, thoughts, and behaviors as understandable within the context of their personal experience. This validation serves as a powerful antidote to the invalidation that so often accompanies trauma, where one's reality and pain are dismissed or ignored, inflicting even deeper wounds.

The individual therapy component within DBT provides an intimate space where clients can peel back the layers of their trauma narrative, exposing the raw edges in a safe and structured environment. The therapeutic alliance becomes a crucible for transformation as clients test new skills and refine them under the attentive guidance of their therapist.

DBT's group skills training component complements individual therapy by immersing clients in a supportive community of peers who share similar struggles. Group sessions offer a collective space where learning is amplified through shared experiences and mutual support, reinforcing the individual's progress.

The role of the therapist in DBT extends beyond that of a mere facilitator; they embody the principle of dialectical thinking, balancing nurturance with challenge, acceptance with the demand for change. The therapist becomes an ally, shaping the therapy to meet the client's needs while adhering to the structured, evidence-based framework that DBT provides.

In the dance of DBT for trauma, phone coaching is yet another step—one that reinforces the therapeutic relationship by providing clients with real-time support when facing challenges outside of therapy sessions. This lifeline fosters a sense of security and continuity, bridging the gap between sessions and everyday life.

Central to the success of DBT for trauma is the therapist's own self-care and awareness. DBT therapists are trained to be mindful of their limits, to seek supervision, and to engage in their own self-care practices, thus ensuring that they bring their best selves to the therapeutic relationship. This focus on the well-being of the therapist creates a replenishing cycle where both client and therapist are supported in their mutual journey toward healing.

As we zero in on DBT's essence for trauma therapy, it's clear that its precision and adaptability make it a robust framework for clients to reconstruct a life stained by trauma. It offers a scaffold upon which persons can rebuild, redesign, and re-engage with life in a way that honors their past while embracing a future abundant with possibility.

DBT for trauma isn't just a clinical approach; it's a testament to the resilience of the human spirit. It champions the power within each individual to step beyond the shadows of their experience into a light that not only shines upon them but also radiates from them, instilling hope and serving as a beacon to others on their own paths to recovery.

In the practice of trauma therapy, DBT stands as a reminder that even amidst the turbulence of our deepest struggles, there lies an opportunity for profound growth and healing. It is an invitation to journey through pain with courage, and arrive at a place where suffering is transformed into strength—a lesson in the alchemy of the human condition.

Exposure Therapies: Prolonged Exposure (PE) and EMDR

As we turn to the potent therapeutic modalities housed under cognitive and behavioral interventions, we delve into two approaches that have transformed the landscape of trauma therapy: Prolonged Exposure (PE) and Eye Movement Desensitization and Reprocessing (EMDR). These evidence-based practices are cornerstones of empowerment, offering clients the means to reclaim their lives from the grasp of trauma.

Prolonged Exposure therapy is a form of cognitive-behavioral therapy specifically designed to help individuals confront their trauma-related memories, feelings, and situations. The core concept behind PE is the principle of habituation - the idea that exposure to a feared object or context reduces the fear response with repeated encounters.

PE consists of four key components: psychoeducation about the nature of trauma and its effects, breathing retraining to manage anxiety, repeated in vivo confrontation with trauma triggers, and imaginal exposure to traumatic memories. Akin to a warrior stepping back into the arena, clients gradually face their fears in a controlled environment, diminishing their power.

The transformation that unfolds through PE is not merely about extinguishing fear; it's about rewriting the narrative that has ensnared the client's identity. By safely revisiting the trauma, individuals can process and integrate the experience, often leading to a significant reduction in PTSD symptoms.

EMDR, on the other hand, employs a unique method of structured therapy that includes a multi-phase process of desensitizing and reprocessing distressing memories. It is innovative in that it does not rely solely on direct exposure or the detailed description of traumatic events. EMDR incorporates bilateral stimulation, typically through guided eye movements, which is believed to mimic the psychological state associated with Rapid Eye Movement (REM) sleep.

Clients undergoing EMDR treatment focus on a traumatic memory while simultaneously experiencing bilateral stimulation that may involve following the therapist's fingers with their eyes or through auditory or tactile stimuli. This process facilitates the reorganization of the traumatic experience within the brain, so it's stored with less distress and becomes a part of a cohesive narrative of the past.

EMDR therapy is guided by the Adaptive Information Processing model, which posits that symptoms arise when experiences are inadequately processed and are thus inadequately integrated into one's overarching life story. Through the phases of EMDR, memories are believed to be digested and stored appropriately, diminishing the symptoms of trauma.

The journey through EMDR is not simply about symptom relief; it is about transformation. As erroneous beliefs forged in trauma are confronted and revised, individuals often experience a powerful sense of freedom. They move forward empowered by an intrinsic resilience that supports their continued growth and healing.

Both PE and EMDR are grounded in structures that promote safety and predictability. For example, in PE, creating a hierarchy of trauma memories facilitates a gradual approach, while EMDR's structured phases ensure a methodical progression through processing.

Safety is of paramount importance when employing these therapies. Preparatory work centers around building strong therapeutic alliances, offering coping strategies, and assessing client readiness. It's imperative for clients not only to face their traumas but to do so feeling supported and capable, thereby enhancing the therapy's efficacy.

Consideration for individual differences is at the heart of exposure therapies. Cultural nuances, personality traits, and co-occurring disorders are factored into the tailored approach for each client. Therapists must be adept at navigating such complexities to foster positive outcomes.

Both PE and EMDR boast impressive empirical evidence supporting their use in treating trauma and PTSD. Numerous studies have demonstrated their effectiveness, helping clients reduce the intensity of their traumatic memories and leading to symptom remission. In many cases, these therapies provide a renewed sense of normalcy and function for survivors of trauma.

As therapists, when guiding clients through the transformative process of PE or EMDR, it is crucial to highlight their intrinsic strength. The act of facing one's traumatic history is a testament to human resilience. Clients are not merely removing symptoms; they are reclaiming their narratives, their autonomy, and their right to peace.

Continuous monitoring of progress and client reactions is an intrinsic part of these therapies. Therapists must be cautious to avoid re-traumatization and attuned to subtle shifts in their clients' readiness and emotional states, adjusting the process as needed to support their therapeutic journey.

Training and competence in these methods are non-negotiables. Because exposure therapies can evoke strong emotional reactions, therapists must possess extensive knowledge and skill. This includes being able to maintain a calm, reassuring presence and the ability to help clients navigate intense emotional experiences.

Lastly, it's important to emphasize that while PE and EMDR are powerful tools, they are part of a broader, integrative treatment plan. Trauma therapy often necessitates a combination of approaches, and these exposure therapies may be interwoven with other modalities to support the overall healing process.

For those embarking on the challenging yet rewarding endeavor of exposure therapy, remember that alongside your clients, you are not just confronting trauma, but forging a path to resilience and healing. Your role is pivotal, possessing the potential to turn the tide in someone's life, guiding them towards liberation from the past and a brighter, trauma-informed future.

Chapter 7:
Narrative and Expressive Therapies

In Chapter 7, "Narrative and Expressive Therapies," we delve deep into the healing power of storytelling and creative expression. In the heart of this transformative chapter, we unlock the cathartic potency of narratives as tools for clients to reshape and reclaim their personal histories marred by trauma. Here, you'll learn how the delicate art of storytelling can be a client's faithful ally, empowering them to author a new chapter in their lives, where they are not just survivors, but heroes of their own epic. We'll explore the intricate corridors of art and movement therapy, where the unspoken sorrows and joys find a vibrant palette and a freeing dance, enabling clients to articulate emotions that words alone cannot convey. Additionally, you'll discover the liberating force of writing and various expressive modalities, where the act of externalizing inner turmoil initiates a transformative journey towards healing. Let's immerse in these profound therapies that inspire, invigorate, and illuminate the uncharted pathways to recovery, guiding those in your care towards a horizon filled with hope and renewed narrative agency.

Transforming Trauma Through Storytelling

In the heart of human connection lies the power of storytelling. It's the thread that weaves the fabric of our collective experience, binding us in understanding, empathy, and ultimately healing. Within the realm of trauma therapy, storytelling emerges not just as a cultural keystone but as a profound therapeutic instrument. The act of narrative construction lends those traumatized the ability to externalize their experiences, offering a bridge from dissonance to coherence.

For individuals who've been silenced by their traumas, storytelling represents a reclaiming of voice. It's an empowering approach that invites them to author their own narratives, rather than being defined by the events that have befallen them. This process involves a delicate balance, navigating the waters of past and present to script a future where traumatic memories are acknowledged yet stripped of their commandeering power.

Storytelling is multilayered when applied to trauma-informed therapy. It allows therapists to help clients organize chaotic experiences into a sequential storyline that can make sense of the senseless. Crafting a narrative goes beyond mere recounting; it's about shaping meaning, gaining insight, and engaging in a process of transformation and identity reformation.

Therapists utilize various methods to elicit stories from their clients, understanding that the journey of recounting trauma can be as arduous as the trauma itself. It's this space that requires utmost sensitivity, where we gently encourage the narration of events while safeguarding the wellbeing of our clients. We must traverse this path with respect for each person's pace and readiness.

Narrative therapy, a pillar in the field, sets the stage for clients to externalize their trauma. The trauma thus becomes a separate entity from the individual—a problem to be dealt with outside of themselves. This distancing can reduce feelings of shame and guilt, as clients recognize that they are not the problem; the trauma is.

As we delve deeper into the storytelling process, we understand its cyclic nature in healing. Each retelling of the traumatic event from the client's perspective can desensitize its impact and diminish its hold.

The narrative, like a book being edited, transforms over time, adopting new perspectives and integrating client strengths and support systems.

The act of storytelling in therapy carries immense cathartic potential, providing a purge of pent-up emotions. Clients experience a release, a form of liberation through the sharing of their pain, which, when held within, can become toxic. In that release is the potential for lightness and a future less burdened by the weight of untold stories.

When tailoring narrative interventions, one must be mindful of the individual's cultural and social contexts. Stories are not just personal; they are filled with the nuances of the client's background, and these distinct cultural narratives play a crucial role in shaping the therapeutic journey. Such awareness ensures that storytelling becomes a culturally attuned pathway to healing.

Through stories, people can not only reclaim their history but also construct a resilient identity. As clients narrate their stories, they discover an inner strength previously unrecognized. This strength becomes a cornerstone of their new self-narrative, one that encompasses survival and the capacity for growth.

Clinicians must bear in mind the vicarious impact of these heavy narratives. As we listen to stories of trauma, we not only bear witness to our clients' pain but also absorb it. Maintaining our objectivity and managing our own emotions is paramount to providing effective treatment and protecting our mental health.

Storytelling is an art, and when it intertwines with the science of therapy, it has the potential to be transformative. As therapists, we are tasked with providing the right environment, prompts, and interventions that facilitate positive re-authoring of traumatic experiences. We must remember that each client is the author of their story, and we are merely the guides providing them with the tools to pen their next chapters.

Integrating storytelling into trauma therapy is a dynamic process. It blends narrative techniques with expressive arts, somatic practices, and cognitive methods, creating a comprehensive approach to healing. This integration acknowledges that the story of trauma resides not only in the mind but also in the body and spirit of the survivor.

Ultimately, transforming trauma through storytelling is about shifting the focus from trauma as pathology to trauma as part of the human experience that requires acknowledgment, support, and integration. It's a powerful testament to the resilience of the human spirit and the transformative capacities of narrative within a safe and supportive therapeutic relationship.

As we progress in the field of trauma therapy, storytelling remains a beacon of hope. It is through the re-authoring of individual narratives that healing permeates, resilience is fortified, and lives are rebuilt. Let us, as therapists, continue to refine our skills in narrative facilitation, honoring the stories of those who seek solace and strength in their journey toward recovery.

In conclusion, storytelling is an indispensable tool in the trauma therapist's toolkit, one that fosters connection, restoration, and empowerment. It goes beyond mere words; it's a process of transformation that can restore broken spirits and breathe life into shattered dreams. We stand as witnesses to the stories of resilience, guiding our clients towards weaving a tale not just of survival, but of thriving in the aftermath of trauma.

Art and Movement Therapy

As we delve into the nuanced approaches under the umbrella of *Narrative and Expressive Therapies*, it's imperative to recognize the transformative power of **Art and Movement Therapy**. Healing from trauma is not only a cognitive endeavor but also a visceral, embodied experience. The languages of art and movement offer unique pathways to expression when words alone may not suffice.

Art therapy has an intrinsic ability to unlock emotional expression and foster healing. It is a dynamic force in rewriting the traumatic narrative without the constraints of verbal communication. *Art and Movement Therapy* engages clients in the creative process to help them externalize inner turmoil, confront difficult emotions, and navigate their trauma with color, shape, and form as their guides.

Movement therapy, alternatively known as dance therapy, utilizes the body's motions to catalyze emotional release and cognitive processing. While trauma can cause a disconnect from one's own body, movement therapy bridges this gap, allowing clients to reclaim their physical space and explore the nuanced stories that their bodies hold.

Incorporating these therapies into practice not only broadens our therapeutic toolkit but demonstrates a deep respect for the individual and unique ways in which people process and express their traumas. Clients are often surprised by the self-discoveries that emerge through their artistic creations and movement sequences.

The nonverbal storytelling facilitated by art can serve as a powerful medium for individuals to represent their experiences. This visual representation becomes a tangible reflection of their inner world, often illuminating paths to insight and understanding that might have otherwise remained obscured. Meanwhile, movement allows for a kinesthetic dialogue between the mind and the body, often revealing subconscious thoughts and memories.

In the safety of the therapeutic space, clients can explore materials and movement without judgment, which can be particularly liberating for those who have felt imprisoned by their traumatic experiences. It's crucial, however, to remain acutely sensitive to the fact that both art and movement can expose vulnerabilities and that a supportive, gentle approach is essential.

One might question how such expressive modalities measure up against more traditional forms of therapy. The evidence suggests that these approaches can reduce symptoms of anxiety, depression, and post-traumatic stress disorder, as well as facilitate improvements in self-esteem and overall well-being.

When integrating **Art and Movement Therapy**, therapists are invited to bear witness to their clients' nonverbal expressions and encourage them to delve into the representations they create. Such therapeutic interactions often reveal metaphors and symbols that can be deciphered and woven into a narrative of recovery.

The therapist's role in this process is multifaceted. While they are a guide and supporter, they also interpret and mirror back the client's nonverbal cues, assisting in the elaboration of their story. This interactive process can help clients understand the links between their past traumas and current behaviors, choices, and emotions, thus facilitating a deeper healing journey.

Additionally, the collaborative nature of **Art and Movement Therapy** fosters a sense of mastery and control, allowing clients to dictate the pace and direction of their therapy. This reinforcement of autonomy is particularly salient for those whose traumas have left them feeling powerless and without a voice.

The versatility of expressive therapies also allows customization to fit individual needs. One session might focus on freeform painting to explore emotional states, while another could involve choreographed movements to address specific body-memory. The therapies are adaptable and can be modified for age, ability, and cultural relevance, ensuring accessibility for all clients.

Success in **Art and Movement Therapy** does not hinge on artistic or dance prowess; the therapeutical value lies in the process rather than the end product. It is about the unfolding narrative, the gradual layering of meaning, and the personal insights gained. Clients are reassured that they are not evaluated on their performance or skill, but encouraged to embrace the therapeutic aspect of creative expression.

Furthermore, group settings can be especially beneficial in these therapies. Group art or movement sessions establish a shared environment where empathy and collective support thrive. It is within this communal space that individuals can bear witness to others' healing journeys and feel less isolated in their own.

Deploying **Art and Movement Therapy** facilitates a holistic approach where trauma survivors can engage in a full spectrum of self-expression. Echoing an essential belief in trauma-informed care, these therapies honor the principle that there are many paths to healing, and each person's journey is honored as unique and valid.

In conclusion, the essence of **Art and Movement Therapy** within the context of trauma-informed care is about creating space for growth, expression, and transformation. These modalities complement narrative approaches, enabling individuals to tell their stories in ways that resonate deeply with their personal experiences. As mental health professionals, embracing these therapies enriches our practices and empowers those we serve, fostering resilience and hope in the face of adversity.

Writing and Other Expressive Modalities

In the realm of healing from trauma, the might of the written word can't be overstated. Through writing, clients find a unique opportunity to express their innermost thoughts and feelings in a format that's at once tangible and alterable. This modality, within the umbrella of narrative and expressive therapies, stands as a testament to the notion that language itself can be a pathway to transformation.

When individuals craft their narratives through writing, they effectively engage in an act of re-authoring their personal histories. It's not merely about reflecting on the facts of their experiences; it's an explorative process that allows them to reframe and potentially come to terms with traumatic events. Writing offers a space where they can take control, experiment with different outcomes, and rebuild their stories with empowered voices.

Let's not forget the versatility of writing as a modality. There is strength in its adaptability, whether it's structured as in narrative therapy, or free-flowing like journaling or poetry. Each form serves a unique purpose, illuminating distinct paths toward healing. In structured writing, the therapist might guide a client to articulate their experience with intention and detail, focusing on coherence and understanding. Alternatively, free-form writing, such as expressive writing, can unlock emotions and thoughts that lie beneath the surface, capturing the raw essence of the person's experience.

Journaling is a particularly powerful practice in trauma therapy. It becomes a private retreat, a safe haven, where one can confront and converse with their traumas without fear of judgment or interruption. Regular journaling nurtures a practice of self-reflection and catharsis that can be liberating for individuals who've felt imprisoned by their traumatic histories. It's a practice that can incrementally build resilience and self-awareness.

Equally compelling is the use of poetry in therapy — a conduit for expression that can bypass the constraints of conventional language. Through metaphor, symbolism, and rhythm, clients can give voice to experiences that might otherwise be unspeakable. The abstract nature of poetry accommodates the complexities of trauma, allowing for healing expressions that prose can't always capture.

Life scripts, another expressive writing technique, allow clients to identify recurring patterns in their lives and consider how these might be rooted in past trauma. Rewriting these scripts can foster a sense of agency, empowering clients to begin changing unhelpful patterns that have held sway over their lives. It's a process of recognizing one's capacity for change, and grasping the pen firmly to do so.

Letter writing, whether to oneself or to others, can also serve as a therapeutic tool. It's a powerful means of giving voice to unspoken words, articulating forgiveness, or asserting one's needs and boundaries. Letters may never be sent, but their creation is an act of symbolic communication that can have profound internal significance.

Beyond solitary writing, the therapeutic application of bibliotherapy — the use of literature as a form of treatment — can tap into the healing power of shared human experiences. Clients may find comfort and insight in the stories of others, seeing reflections of their own journey in the narratives of characters navigating adversity. This can sometimes make one's own struggles feel less isolating and more universal.

Digital storytelling, too, has emerged as a contemporary expressive modality. Integrating multimedia elements with personal narratives, it allows clients to tell their stories using voice, images, and music. The multisensory experience of creating and sharing a digital story can be immensely cathartic and validating, especially for those whose trauma has muted their perceived ability to communicate effectively.

The rise of blogging and social media as platforms for storytelling introduces another layer of complexity to narrative expression. They offer a public domain for sharing and collective engagement, which can be both empowering and daunting. The act of making one's story public can be a profound step toward reclaiming power over that story, yet it must be approached with caution, ensuring readiness and emotional safety.

Despite the therapeutic potential of writing and other expressive modalities, practitioners must be conscious of the potential for re-traumatization. Writing about trauma can sometimes surface intense emotions and triggering memories. It's essential that therapists provide a safe, supportive space and are prepared to help clients manage any distress that arises. Real healing happens within a framework of safety and trust; writing is no exception to this rule.

As therapists integrate writing into their practice, it's crucial to remember that these are not prescribed activities with guaranteed outcomes but rather fluid interventions. Flexibility and attunement to the individual's needs are vital. The timing, the type of writing, the frequency — all should be tailored to support the client's unique therapeutic journey.

Writing and other expressive modalities aren't just clinical tools; they are powerful extensions of the client's voice. Harnessing these techniques can become life-altering, carving paths to understanding, acceptance, and, ultimately, transformation. These modes of expression encourage the internalization of a narrative of survival and strength, which can be the cornerstone of reconstructing an identity that's been fragmented by trauma.

In closing, as practitioners empower clients to navigate their healing process, they do so with a deep recognition of the sanctity of each word written and every story told. It's a partnership, a dance of narrative reconstruction, where the therapist's role is to provide the rhythm for the client's steps, guiding them toward empowerment and the reclamation of their story, one word at a time.

Chapter 8:
Group Therapy and Community Support

As we journey deeper into the healing landscape of trauma therapy, we find that the collective heartbeats within group therapy and the broad embrace of community support offer pivotal pathways to recovery. Imagine a space where the shared stories and empathic resonance of multiple individuals create a tapestry of healing, where one feels less alone in their struggles and more connected through their collective journey. Group dynamics unfold with precision and care, guided by facilitators who understand the nuanced ebb and flow of traumatic experiences. The role of these therapeutic groups isn't merely to foster a sense of belonging but to cultivate a transformative environment where reflection, connection, and growth can occur simultaneously. Beyond the confidential walls of the therapy room, engaging community resources and support networks becomes a vital extension of support, as it reinforces the client's resilience and encourages integration with wider systems of care. Within this chapter, the potent interplay between group therapy and community support is explored—reminding us that our social interconnectedness serves as both a buffer and a bridge in the profound healing process of trauma.

The Power of Group Dynamics in Healing

As we delve into the intricacies of group therapy and community support, it's important to highlight an undeniable force within this therapeutic milieu: the power of group dynamics in healing. The collective energy that arises from shared experiences, stories, and struggles can't be replicated in individual therapy, and harnessing this force becomes instrumental in steering individuals towards recovery and growth.

In the context of trauma, where isolation often exacerbates suffering, the group becomes a sanctuary for connection and understanding. The sense of belonging that emerges within a group has a profound impact on an individual's healing journey, reminding participants that they're not alone in their struggles. In a group, members find their reflections in each other's narratives, providing validation and normalizing their emotional experiences.

Group dynamics work on various levels to aid healing. Firstly, camaraderie fosters resilience. Witnessing others grappling with similar issues instills hope and a belief in the possibility of overcoming personal hurdles. As members share accomplishments or break-throughs, it acts as a catalyst for others. The shared celebration of progress bolsters the group's morale and drives collective triumph.

Furthermore, the safety net provided by the group encourages risk-taking in the form of emotional vulnerability. In a well-facilitated group, individuals learn to lower their psychological defenses, a process that is both cathartic and crucial for working through traumatic material. The dynamic of mutual support allows for the expression of emotions and fears that might remain unspoken in other contexts.

Feedback within a group can be transformative. Receiving comments from peers, who have no other agenda than healing, often resonates differently than feedback from a therapist. This is because group members speak a shared language rooted in lived experience, which can penetrate through walls of resistance and denial, illuminating blind spots with remarkable grace.

Importantly, the microcosm of a therapy group simulates a larger societal framework, granting members the chance to practice new behaviors in a controlled environment. Social skills, conflict resolution, and assertiveness can all be honed within the group setting, informed by instant feedback and support.

The group dynamic also nurtures the development of empathy. By being exposed to a diversity of trauma narratives, members expand their own emotional range. They learn to hold space for others' pain, which in turn, teaches them how to approach their own suffering with compassion rather than judgment or avoidance.

The role of the therapist in this delicate ecosystem is to guide and foster the group's therapeutic potential. A skilled facilitator paves the way for positive group dynamics by establishing boundaries, promoting inclusivity, and ensuring psychological safety. This cultivation of a positive group culture is as crucial as any intervention delivered in a one-on-one session.

Despite the numerous benefits of group dynamics, it's imperative to recognize the careful balance required to maintain its healing power. Challenges such as group conflict, dominance by certain members, or sub-grouping can diminish the therapeutic value if not addressed promptly and effectively. Therapists need to remain vigilant and agile, ready to intervene when the group's equilibrium is at risk.

Let us not underestimate the role of collective healing rituals within group therapy. Ceremonies, shared practices, and group traditions build a strong alliance and identity. They knit the fabric of the group tighter, offering a powerful antidote to the disconnection wrought by trauma.

Peer modeling within the group becomes a powerful vehicle for change. Seeing others actively engage in recovery behaviors and self-care can be inspirational. It provides tangible proof of coping strategies and resilience in action, offering a roadmap for others to follow.

Accountability is an additional gift group therapy bestows upon its members. Knowing that the group is a witness to one's commitments can fortify an individual's resolve to make changes. This collective accountability can be a crucial factor in maintaining progress and preventing relapse.

As part of an integrative approach to trauma therapy, group dynamics offer an interweaving of relationship dynamics that can do more than just educate or build skills. It forges a community that collectively engages with the very core of trauma healing: relationship and connection.

Group therapy, when well-executed, cultivates a culture of growth, learning, and healing that is greater than the sum of its parts. It serves as a testament to the human capacity for resilience and the transformative power of shared healing journeys. The dynamic interplay between group members creates a rich tapestry of interpersonal experiences that facilitate deep insight, profound change, and most importantly, hope for a future unhindered by the burdens of trauma.

In embracing group therapy and community support, mental health professionals are not only leveraging the power of group dynamics but are also recognizing the inherent social nature of human beings. We're designed to heal in the company of others, finding strength and solace in shared stories and the collective pursuit of wellbeing. As we continue to explore and implement trauma-informed care, let's remember that the group's potential to heal is a potent force, one that can significantly contribute to the restoration of those we aim to serve.

Facilitating Trauma-Informed Group Therapy

In the realm of healing, group therapy can be a potent catalyst for transformation, particularly when dealing with the impacts of trauma.

Its efficacy lies in its collective nature; allowing individuals to find solace, support, and a shared space for recovery. As facilitators, it's essential to approach trauma-informed group therapy with sensitivity, structure, empathy, and adaptability. Let's delve into the mechanisms that make this therapeutic approach resonate with survivors, fostering resilience and fostering change.

The first step in facilitating trauma-informed group therapy is creating a foundation of safety. Safety is paramount, as it allows for the vulnerabilities of trauma to be explored within an environment of acceptance. Establish a clear set of guidelines and protocols, which serve both as boundaries and as sources of reassurance. Ground rules that prioritize confidentiality and mutual respect are not merely procedural; they are the cornerstones upon which healing can begin.

Remember that trauma interrupts a person's narrative, leaving fragments that may feel disconnected or overwhelming. Group therapy aims to mend these tattered narratives through shared storytelling. Empower your group members to speak their truths, all the while ensuring that each voice is heard and validated. Listening is as healing as sharing, and as a facilitator, model active, empathetic listening to foster a culture of understanding within the group.

At times, verbal exchange alone may not suffice to convey the complex emotions associated with trauma. Thus, integrating expressive therapies such as art or movement can be instrumental. These methods offer alternative avenues of expression, giving form to internal experiences that words might fail to encapsulate. Providing a variety of expressive outlets recognizes the diverse ways individuals process and express their trauma.

Connection is the lifeblood of group therapy. In a trauma-informed setting, seek to reinforce the human need for connection and the longing for a community of peers who empathize with each other's journeys. Encourage collaborative activities that build cohesion, such as group projects or shared goals, as these endeavors foster a sense of belonging and common purpose.

Mindfulness and grounding techniques are invaluable tools within your facilitator's toolbox. They serve to anchor participants in the present, guiding the group away from turbulent memories or anxieties about the future. Teach these techniques early on and revisit them frequently, making mindfulness a foundational practice of the group's routine.

Expect and plan for emotional variability within the group. Trauma responses can be unpredictable, surfacing in myriad ways from tears to anger, withdrawal to confrontation. As a facilitator, maintain a stable presence, navigating these waters with a steady hand, and equipping the group to handle these reactions with compassion and without judgment.

Trust-building exercises are another critical component. Trust may have been shattered by past traumas, and rebuilding it within the group context takes time and deliberate effort. Create opportunities for small victories of trust, such as dependability exercises or paired sharing, to gradually fortify the group's confidence in each other.

As the group develops, focus on resilience and strengths rather than solely on vulnerabilities. Remind the members of their inherent capacities to cope and thrive, underscoring the progress they've already made. This not only recognizes their journey but also propels them towards continued healing and growth.

Recognize the importance of individual pacing. While the group moves together on a shared trajectory, each member's path is unique. Some may advance quickly, while others require more time to process and engage with the material. Be flexible and patient, acknowledging that healing does not follow a linear timeline.

Facilitating trauma-informed group therapy also means being culturally attuned. You're not merely guiding a group through trauma recovery; you're navigating the nuances of diverse backgrounds, values, beliefs, and worldviews. Ensure that your approach is inclusive and respectful of the cultural dimensions that each group member brings to the session.

Conflict may arise in such an intimate setting. Handling disagreements empathetically, while ensuring that each member feels seen and heard, maintains the cohesion of the group. Encourage open dialogue about conflicts when they occur, using them as opportunities for learning and deeper understanding.

Document the group's journey, both for your professional record and to celebrate the milestones you reach together. This shared history becomes a testament to the group's work, a narrative of collective triumph over adversity. Reviewing this record not only assists in tracking progress but also reinforces the group's achievements.

Self-disclosure from the therapist can at times be helpful in establishing a reciprocal and authentic environment. However, it is important to disclose selectively and mindfully, ensuring that the focus remains on the clients and that the disclosure serves the group's therapeutic goals.

Finally, reflection and closure are vital in each session and throughout the therapy process. Help the group reflect on their individual and collective experiences, highlighting insights gained and reinforcing the sense of journeying together. As the group therapy process culminates, facilitate a thoughtful and meaningful closure that honors the shared experiences and individual contributions to the group's healing process.

Facilitating trauma-informed group therapy is a journey that requires diligence, empathy, and unwavering commitment. As you pilot this vessel through the healing waters, remember that each session is a step towards empowering survivors to reclaim their narratives. You are a guide, a witness, and a companion in their journey—a response-bility that is deeply honorable and profoundly transformative.

Engaging Community Resources and Support Networks

As we delve deeper into the pivotal role of group therapy and community support for those who've lived through trauma, it becomes essential to recognize the expansive ecosystem of potential allies and resources at our disposal. The philosophy behind this is not merely a matter of convenience but of holistic healing. Community resources and support networks can play a transformative role in reinforcing the work done within the therapeutic setting and fostering a sense of belonging and connection for clients striving to navigate the aftermath of traumatic experiences.

In the journey toward healing, clients often seek more than just individual therapy; they need the richness of diverse perspectives and the support that comes from collective wisdom. The establishment of a network of organizations, services, and groups can act as an integral extension of the therapeutic process, where clients can continue to learn, grow, and find support outside the confines of the therapy room. Engaging community resources, therefore, transcends traditional therapy and embraces an ecological framework for recovery, one where external supports and resources become an integral part of the healing landscape.

One of the first steps in connecting clients to community resources is to maintain an up-to-date and comprehensive list of local support groups, non-profit organizations, advocacy services, and recreational activities that are trauma-informed. For clients, knowing that there are group gatherings and activities specifically geared toward individuals with similar experiences can ease the isolation and stigmatization often associated with trauma. Moreover, active participation in such groups can help to contextualize their own experiences through the stories and insights of others.

To ensure that clients receive the best possible referral, therapists should become familiar with these community resources firsthand. This might involve visiting support groups, liaising with organizers, and continually assessing the quality and effectiveness of these resources. Doing so underpins the credibility of the therapist and validates the significance of each recommended resource. It's not enough to simply provide a pamphlet; the therapist's genuine belief in the resource's value is impactful and motivates client engagement.

Incorporating community resources into treatment plans demands a tailored approach. Each client's history, cultural identity, and preferences should guide the selection of appropriate resources. Therapists can facilitate introductions and even accompany clients to new groups or events to ease the transition and bolster their confidence in trying new avenues of support. This active facilitation demonstrates empathy and dedication, showing clients that they are not alone in this broader healing journey.

Engagement with community resources is a dynamic process, with clients' needs and the availability of resources evolving over time. Thus, therapists should employ an ongoing assessment and feedback loop with their clients in relation to these external supports. What works for one client at a certain stage of their healing may not suit another, or the same client might outgrow a particular group or activity. Regular check-ins allow for adjustments and continued personalization of support strategies.

Peer-to-peer support is another critical facet of community engagement. Peer-support programs, which empower individuals who have experienced trauma themselves to support others, endorse the philosophy that healing can be found through mutual help. In these peer dynamics, clients often encounter role models who inspire hope and provide living proof that recovery is not only possible but within reach.

For some clients, engaging with resource centers that provide practical assistance with housing, employment, legal issues, or education can be instrumental in their recovery process. These resource centers can alleviate the external pressures that, when left unaddressed, may exacerbate the emotional and psychological distress of their trauma. Therapists should actively explore these options and provide information and referrals to ensure that clients' basic needs are not neglected.

Beyond formal resources, communities are reservoirs of informal supports that can play a sizable role in the healing process. Encouraging clients to participate in community events, such as local fairs, public lectures, or volunteer activities, can foster a sense of connection and purpose. The gradual rebuilding of social networks in safe, structured environments contributes significantly to the regaining of trust and the reconstruction of a supportive social fabric.

Collaboration between therapists and community leaders can also yield new opportunities for clients. Hosting community workshops, awareness events, or participating in local councils and coalitions dedicated to trauma-informed initiatives are ways in which therapists can advocate for their clients and influence broader systemic change.

When engaging with communities, confidentiality remains sacrosanct. Therapists and clients must navigate the public aspect of community engagement with care, ensuring that clients' rights to privacy are upheld and that participation in groups or events does not inadvertently expose sensitive information. This might involve discussing ground rules prior to the engagement or seeking closed, anonymous groups where confidentiality is a shared value.

In our increasingly digital world, online communities have emerged as a significant adjunct to local venues. Virtual support groups, forums, and social media platforms allow for connections that transcend geographic barriers. Therapists should guide clients in finding reputable online resources and advocate for digital literacy to ensure that clients can engage safely and effectively.

The therapeutic alliance remains a fundamental cornerstone of trauma therapy, yet we cannot ignore the exponential potential for healing that lies within the collective strength of community resources and support networks. Hence, our role as mental health professionals extends into the realm of community connectors—advising, guiding, and walking alongside clients as they traverse the road to recovery beyond our office doors.

Engagement with community resources and support networks is a testament to a core realization: healing from trauma is as much an individual quest as it is a communal endeavor. By nurturing this alliance between individual therapy and community resources, we provide our clients with the very best chance for a well-rounded, sustainable recovery, touching lives and transforming communities in the process.

In summary, it's our privileged task to shine a light on paths that lead our clients not only towards recovery but towards a sense of kinship and societal integration. To wield the power of community in the service of healing is to weave a richer tapestry of support—an approach that acknowledges and cherishes the profound interconnectedness of our human journey.

Chapter 9:
Trauma in Special Populations

Building on the foundation of trauma-informed care, we now turn our attention to the unique challenges and needs of special populations. In this chapter, we delve into the nuanced landscape of trauma therapy with particularly vulnerable groups: children and adolescents, older adults, and those from marginalized and oppressed communities. Each of these groups carries distinct histories and faces specific barriers that require tailored approaches. The legacy of trauma's impact on these populations may be profound, and thus, sensitivity to their specific circumstances, resilience, and potential for growth is paramount. We'll explore how to craft approaches that not only address but honor their unique life stories, fostering a sense of safety and empowerment that is both healing and transformative. Our goal is to illuminate the path to healing, ensuring that every individual, irrespective of age, background, or societal position, has access to the compassionate and skilled support they need to reclaim their narrative and embrace a future with hope and strength.

Trauma Therapy with Children and Adolescents

As mental health practitioners, we encounter myriad expressions of the human condition throughout our practice. Among the most delicate paths we tread is the one that involves the hearts and minds of children and adolescents who have witnessed or experienced trauma. When working with this vulnerable population, therapeutic intervention involves not only skill but also profound sensitivity.

Childhood and adolescence are fundamental stages of development. Trauma during these formative years can significantly alter the course of emotional and psychological growth, sometimes with lasting repercussions into adulthood. Even as their bodies heal from any physical injuries, the invisible wounds nested within their psyche often require an attuned approach to unearth and mend.

The term "trauma" envelops a range of experiences—from one-time incidents to ongoing, chronic abuse or neglect. With children and adolescents, it's imperative to recognize that their lack of life experience and still-developing brains make them particularly sensitive to trauma. Their responses to fear and stress can become deeply embedded, calling for a gentle yet deliberate method of therapy.

Creating a space of safety is the foundational stone upon which all trauma therapy rests, particularly with younger populations. Their perceptions of the world are still forming, often around the traumatic experiences they've had. It's our job to reconstruct that perception to one that sees the world as a place where they can feel secure and thrive.

Building trust is an essential component of trauma work with children and adolescents. Developing a solid therapeutic relationship is more than a protocol—it's an art, one that requires us to lean into our own reservoirs of empathy and patience. Each session can be a step toward repairing the fractures within a young spirit, calling for you to celebrate small victories as milestones of progress.

Engaging in therapeutic play can be especially efficacious. Through the lens of play, younger individuals can express thoughts and feelings that might otherwise remain concealed. It's not simply about the toys or games—it's about creating a medium through which they can explore and understand their trauma narratives in a safe and controlled environment.

In conjunction with play, expressive therapies such as art, movement, and music allow for the non-verbal expression of emotions. These tactile and multisensory experiences can be powerful conduits for children and adolescents to release pent-up emotions and begin to articulate their innermost experiences without the demand for verbal precision.

Cognitive-behavioral strategies ought to be adapted for youthful minds, ensuring that concepts such as cognitive restructuring are presented in a manner that's both comprehensible and relatable. We need to speak their language, metaphorically and sometimes literally, to effectively guide them through reframing negative thought patterns.

One cannot overstate the importance of involving caregivers and families in the therapeutic process. A systemic approach, recognizing that children exist within a network of relationships, is crucial. When appropriate, family therapy brings to the fore the dynamics that might either exacerbate or alleviate the youngster's trauma responses.

Developmental sensitivity is a guiding principle in trauma therapy with children and adolescents. Therapies need to be tailored not just to the individual's unique experiences of trauma but also to their developmental stage. The same traumatic event can impact a five-year-old very differently from a fifteen-year-old, requiring different approaches and interventions.

Adolescence is a time of identity formation, and trauma can distort this process. For teens, the therapeutic space can serve as a crucible for forging a sense of self that integrates their experiences without being defined by them. The therapist's role expands to one of a witness and a guide through the murky waters of self-discovery post-trauma.

Exposure therapies, such as Eye Movement Desensitization and Reprocessing (EMDR), can be adapted for the younger population, albeit with care and creativity. These interventions help in processing traumatic memories by accessing the brain's inherent capacity to move toward healing, but always within the context of what is suitable for a child or teenager.

It's important to remember that resilience is not an inexhaustible resource. Childhood and adolescence come with a natural pliancy, and yet, this should not be mistaken for an unlimited ability to bounce back from traumatic events. We are tasked with nurturing and fostering resilience, acting as both catalysts and custodians of their innate strength.

To support growth and healing, we must also advocate for the needs of our young clients in their broader life contexts, such as schools and communities. They should not have to navigate their educational and social environments burdened by unresolved trauma. Instead, they deserve to be met with understanding and accommodations that recognize their unique challenges.

Finally, let us be agents of hope. While we guide children and adolescents through the shadowed valleys of their trauma, let's illuminate paths of possibility and renewal. By instilling hope, we not only aim to help heal the wounds of the past but also to empower our young clients to envision and work towards a future bright with promise.

Addressing Trauma in Older Adults

In our journey to understand and support those who have experienced trauma, we must turn our attention to older adults—a population that may carry a lifetime of traumatic experiences, which manifest uniquely and require tailored therapeutic interventions.

For older adults, trauma often exists as a tapestry woven through a long life, where threads of historical events, personal losses, physical challenges, and societal changes intertwine. As practitioners, recognizing the multiplicity of these traumas and their potential late-life resurgence is paramount to our therapeutic approach.

When addressing trauma in older adults, it's critical to consider the unique context of aging. With age, personal resilience can be both tempered and tested, leading to a complexity in responses to past and present traumas. It's not uncommon for earlier traumatic events to resurface as one encounters the vulnerabilities that come with aging.

Older adults might contend with the trauma brought on by isolation, the loss of loved ones, or the erosion of their own physical and cognitive functions. Such events can retrigger past traumas, and unlike their youthful counterparts, older adults may face these challenges amid a shrinking social support network.

In working with this population, we must emphasize validation and empathy. Validation assures them that their feelings and experiences are real and worthy of attention—even if these events occurred decades ago. Creating a therapeutic environment that resonates with empathy enables them to voice their pain without fear of judgment.

Therapeutic strategies must be molded with sensitivity to the physical and cognitive capabilities of older adults. For some, traditional talk therapy may become strenuous; therefore, employing shorter sessions and incorporating mindfulness and relaxation techniques can be especially beneficial. Using life review interventions can also provide a powerful platform for processing past events and finding meaning in one's life narrative.

Another quintessential consideration is the presence of cognitive decline. Dementia and memory issues might complicate the process of trauma work, potentially obscuring the capacity to engage in certain therapeutic modalities. Thus, therapy must be adapted with a focus on present-moment experiences and emotion regulation techniques that do not solely rely on recall accuracy.

Intergenerational trauma presents yet another layer for consideration. Older adults may carry the weight of traumas relayed from forebears or themselves have been the conduit of such legacies. Therapy may become a space where these inheritances are unraveled and faced with the same courage with which they have been borne.

Integration of somatic therapies can be particularly helpful for older adults, recalibrating the connection between body and mind. Gentle, body-oriented practices support the idea that healing is not bounded by age and that even a body weathered by time can move towards tranquility and away from traumatic stress.

Older adults might face pragmatic challenges, such as transportation or mobility issues, which can impede their access to therapy. Being cognizant of these barriers leads us to creative solutions: providing home-based therapy, using telehealth platforms, or coordinating with local community services to bridge these gaps.

At the core of trauma work with older adults is the principle of empowerment. Allowing them to assert control over their story and their healing process honors their autonomy and leverages their intrinsic strength. It's a journey that acknowledges the multiplicity of their trauma while nurturing the possibility of post-traumatic growth and wisdom.

End-of-life concerns can surface during therapy, bringing forth anxieties about mortality and legacy. The clinical space can transform into a sanctuary where these existential questions are met with compassion and respect, facilitating a process where the older individual can confront and make peace with such concerns.

Cultural sensitivity remains vital in working with older adults. Each individual's cultural background will influence their perception of and response to trauma. As such, therapy must be grounded in an understanding of these cultural factors and how they contribute to the client's experience of trauma and healing.

Collaboration with other care providers, such as physicians, nurses, and social workers, ensures a holistic approach to the older adult's well-being. By incorporating different perspectives and areas of expertise, we create a network of care surrounding the individual that can address the multifaceted nature of their needs.

In summation, treating trauma in older adults demands an approach that is as nuanced as the lives they've lived. It's an endeavor that asks us to weave empathy, respect, and adaptability into every interaction, honoring the resilience and the vulnerabilities of the aging spirit. As we offer solace and understanding, we must always remember that it is never too late for healing to commence and for peace to be attained. Let us be the embodiment of hope for our older clients, as we accompany them on their path toward resolution and tranquility.

Considerations for Marginalized and Oppressed Groups

Healing from trauma is not a one-size-fits-all journey—it's essential to recognize that the paths to recovery are as unique as the individuals walking them. When we consider the experiences of marginalized and oppressed groups, the lens through which we view and interpret trauma must be multifaceted, amplifying empathy and a deep respect for diversity.

Within these communities, trauma doesn't exist in isolation; it intertwines with the systemic barriers, societal bias, and historical oppression that can perpetuate and exacerbate the psychological wounds. This intersectionality of trauma demands that we, as therapists and advocates for mental health, prepare ourselves with an encompassing understanding and skills that are sensitive to the unique circumstances faced by marginalized individuals.

One significant aspect to acknowledge is the historical trauma that affects many communities. This form of trauma is carried across generations and can perpetuate a cycle of adversity that's challenging to break. Understanding the historical context of one's trauma is essential in constructing a therapy approach that doesn't just recognize the present suffering but also the echoes of the past that continue to reverberate.

Stigmatization and discrimination are stark realities that can lead to a compounded experience of trauma. Marginalized groups often encounter barriers in accessing appropriate mental health care, which can be laden with biases or a lack of cultural competence. The therapist's role extends beyond the therapy room—it's about advocating for social justice and reform to reduce these barriers to care.

To foster healing environments, therapeutic approaches must embrace inclusivity. Cultural humility is a lifelong commitment that entails recognizing one's own cultural biases and actively engaging in self-reflection. It's about creating a partnership where the therapist isn't the expert on the client's experience but a collaborative participant in their healing journey.

Language is a powerful tool, and using inclusive, supportive language that respects individuals' identities and experiences is paramount. In therapy, every word counts, and even well-intended language can be harmful if not chosen carefully. The onus is on therapists to educate themselves on evolving terminologies that honor and validate the identities and experiences of the clients they serve.

Safety within therapeutic relationships is not just physical but emotional and psychological. Creating a haven for vulnerable discussions means understanding the fears, resistance, and guardedness that marginalized clients may bring into therapy. Trust has to be built and efforts must be made to dismantle the power dynamics that are often present in the therapeutic relationship.

Intersectionality plays a vital role in understanding client experiences. Marginalized individuals often navigate multiple intersecting identities, all of which can impact the way they experience and respond to trauma. Therapists must move away from a myopic lens and instead view the entity of their client's world through a kaleidoscope of intersecting factors to truly address their needs.

Empowerment is a foundational goal in trauma therapy, but empowerment without awareness of one's social reality is incomplete. The therapeutic intervention must marry empowerment with practical strategies that equip clients to navigate the societal structures that may continue to oppress them even as they heal.

Stereotypes and myths about resilience can also impact the therapeutic process. While it's commonly believed that hardship breeds resilience, this is an oversimplification that can lead to misjudging the support needed by marginalized clients. Resilience should not be an expectation or a prerequisite for compassion and aid—it should be nurtured and supported through therapy.

Accessibility is about more than just creating ramps or providing interpreter services. It's about ensuring that mental health services are socioeconomically accessible, that they're offered in spaces where marginalized individuals feel welcome, and that they're delivered by professionals who reflect the diversity of the community they serve.

Collaboration with community resources is essential. Many marginalized groups have established networks of support that understand their particular challenges. Therapists should be proactive in connecting with these resources to ensure a holistic approach that bridges individual therapy with community support.

Self-advocacy skills are part of the therapeutic process. While therapy often focuses on individual healing, equipping clients with the skills to advocate for their needs and rights in broader society is a powerful tool in transforming trauma into agency.

The inclusive therapeutic approach also involves accountability. Therapists must be willing to recognize and address their mistakes, biases, and areas where they lack knowledge. Ongoing education and peer consultation are key to maintaining a practice that is truly sensitive to the needs of marginalized and oppressed groups.

Lastly, hope is an unwavering ally in the journey to healing. Instilling hope is not about offering empty assurances; it's about recognizing the strength in survival, the potential for change, and the collective effort required to shape a future where trauma doesn't define one's life. It is within this space of optimism accompanied by action that true healing begins to flourish.

Chapter 10:
Pharmacological Interventions and Collaboration with Psychiatrists

A s we dive into the merits and considerations of pharmacological interventions in trauma therapy, Chapter 10 aims to enlighten you on the symbiosis between therapeutic approaches and medication. Tailoring treatment to each individual's needs, we recognize that, sometimes, the path to healing includes psychopharmacology as an adjunct to traditional therapy methods. In these pages, you will come to understand the various medications commonly administered to alleviate the symptoms of trauma, and how they can be integrated effectively into a holistic treatment plan. Establishing a collaborative partnership with psychiatrists is imperative, ensuring that as mental health professionals, we navigate the nuances of pharmacotherapy with skill and care. This collaborative spirit promotes a continuity of care that is both seamless and transparent, ensuring that our clients receive the support they need without falling through the cracks of the healthcare system. You'll learn to balance these interventions with an empathetic, informed approach, weighing benefits and potential risks, and thus empower those we serve in their journey to reclaim their lives from the shadows of trauma.

Medications Commonly Used in Trauma Treatment

As our journey through understanding the multifaceted nature of trauma treatment continues, it's vital to lean into the realm of pharmacological interventions. The careful use of medication can be a cornerstone in holistic trauma therapy, offering a steadying hand to those whose lives have been disrupted by psychological tremors.

When we speak of medications in the context of trauma treatment, it's imperative to recognize that these are tools, not cures. They are designed to alleviate symptoms, provide relief, and enable individuals to engage more fully in therapeutic processes. Various classes of medications are employed to target different symptom clusters and assist in specific areas of need.

Antidepressants, for instance, are often the first line of pharmacological intervention. Selective serotonin reuptake inhibitors (SSRIs), and serotonin-norepinephrine reuptake inhibitors (SNRIs) are frequently prescribed to mitigate symptoms of depression and anxiety, common companions of traumatic stress.

Antidepressants serve to balance chemical messengers in our brains, helping to temper the emotional fluctuations and intrusive thoughts that can impair the journey towards healing. Remember, their effectiveness can be a beacon for some, illuminating a less burdened path forward.

Benzodiazepines may also flirt with the landscape of trauma treatment, offering rapid relief of acute anxiety and agitation. However, these are prescribed with caution due to their potential for dependency and are generally considered a short-term intervention. The relief they provide can offer a window of serenity, allowing those in the throes of traumatic stress to regain a sense of control.

Additionally, mood stabilizers can carve out their niche in the tapestry of trauma care, especially when individuals wrestle with elements of dysregulation or experience symptoms akin to those seen in bipolar disorders. By providing an anchor for emotional highs and lows, mood stabilizers support a steady sail through stormy seas.

Antipsychotic medications might also claim a role, particularly at low doses for those grappling with dissociation or intense, unshakable trauma-related imagery or flashbacks. They work to quiet the haunting echoes of past experiences, granting a more peaceful presence.

In the repertoire of medicinal agents, one mustn't overlook prazosin. Originally used to treat high blood pressure, it has been a revelation for some individuals with PTSD, specifically targeting nightmares and sleep disturbances. The sanctity of restful sleep cannot be understated; it's the golden time our brains and bodies heal.

Additionally, the landscape of trauma treatment sometimes includes the use of beta-blockers. These medications can attenuate the physical symptoms of anxiety, such as palpitations and trembling, acting as a dam against the swell of somatic responses.

For those whose trauma is intertwined with substance use, medications like naltrexone can offer support. By blocking opioid receptors, they reduce cravings and the rewarding effects of substances, making it easier for individuals to maintain sobriety during the peaks and valleys of healing.

Considering the tapestry of trauma and its diverse presentations, there's no one-size-fits-all when it comes to medication. Collaborating with prescribers is a dance that requires steps of open communication, shared expertise, and mutual respect for each individual's unique needs.

While navigating the waters of pharmacological interventions, mental health professionals must stay abreast of the most current, evidence-based practices and research. Furthermore, staying informed about how medications interact with each other and with various therapeutic approaches is key to safeguarding the well-being of those we serve.

In this delicate balance, psychoeducation about medications becomes a responsibility for practitioners. Informing clients about possible side effects, correct usage, and expected timelines for medication effects fosters a sense of agency and aids compliance – both crucial elements in the healing process.

Connection and communication with prescribing psychiatrists thus become not just beneficial, but necessary. Ensuring that all parties are aligned in goals and strategies creates a cohesive support network around the person at the center of this journey, magnifying the potential for transformation.

Let us remember that while medications can be a pivotal part of the treatment plan, they are but one piece of a larger mosaic. Holistic healing requires an integration of approaches; the role medications play is supportive, creating space for therapeutic breakthroughs and personal growth.

In closing this section, it's essential to hold space for the fact that the use of medication, when thoughtfully applied, can be transformative. It's not about numbing or silencing the echoes of the past but about cultivating enough stillness to engage with our internal landscapes. We tread with reverence and care, knowing that each step taken with our clients on this pharmacological path is a step towards reclaiming their lives from the shadows of trauma.

Coordinating Care Between Therapists and Prescribers

In the management of trauma, there are moments where the intersection of therapy and pharmacology becomes not just beneficial but essential. As mental health professionals, our primary concern is the holistic well-being of our clients, a goal that often necessitates collaboration with prescribers, such as psychiatrists, to form a united front against the effects of trauma. Understanding our pivotal role in this partnership is a cornerstone of effective trauma treatment.

At the foundation of effectively coordinating care between therapists and prescribers is clear, open, and consistent communication. Therapists have a unique insight into their clients' daily struggles, progress, and setbacks. It is imperative that we share these observations with prescribers, who can then make informed medication decisions that are congruent with therapeutic goals.

To facilitate collaboration, therapists and prescribers must develop shared objectives for patient outcomes. This partnership is underpinned by mutual respect for each other's expertise. The prescriber's specialized knowledge of psychopharmacology complements the therapist's understanding of psychological processes, trauma's manifestations, and coping strategies employed by the client.

Engaging in regular consultations with prescribers allows therapists to articulate changes in the client's mood, behaviors, and symptoms, which may signal a need for medication adjustments. Likewise, prescribers can provide crucial updates on a client's medication regimen, side-effect profiles, and adherence, which can have significant implications for therapy.

Consent is a pivotal component of successful collaboration. Clients must give permission for their therapist and prescriber to share relevant information. As therapists, we are duty-bound to ensure clients understand the benefits of allowing such a dialogue to occur, emphasizing that it is in service of their recovery.

It is essential to create a systematic approach to coordinating care. This could include regular interprofessional meetings, setting up secure communication channels, or having joint sessions with the client when appropriate. Ensuring that both therapist and prescriber have a mutual understanding and agreement on methods of communication is important for seamless collaboration.

When collaboration is effective, the therapist can assist in the monitoring and management of any pharmacotherapy side effects, which can include physiological changes that might also influence emotional and psychological well-being. Knowledge of these potential side effects arms therapists with the ability to better support their clients and communicate concerns with prescribers promptly.

Another core aspect of coordinating care is the formulation and continuous updating of a treatment plan. This shared document aligns both therapeutic interventions and pharmacological strategies, adjusting as the client evolves through their healing journey. It serves as a living reflection of the client's progress and a roadmap for both therapists and prescribers.

In the context of trauma, it is worth acknowledging that the course of treatment is rarely linear. Therapists and prescribers should be prepared to adapt their approaches to the ebb and flow of the healing process. Flexibility and an open mindset, grounded in the shared goal of client recovery, is essential for adapting to the complexities of trauma treatment.

Cultural competence is another key consideration—both therapists and prescribers must be sensitive to how a client's cultural background may influence their perspectives on medication and therapy. This understanding can lead to more tailored and accepted treatment protocols that honor the individual's cultural beliefs and values.

Education is a role that both therapists and prescribers must embrace. Clients can feel overwhelmed by the complexity of their treatment plans or have concerns about pharmacotherapy. Demystifying these aspects with clear, empathetic discussions empowers clients to take an active role in their treatment, fostering a sense of agency that is critical for trauma recovery.

Documentation is also paramount in collaborative care. Secure record-keeping of shared plans, updates, and assessments ensures that both the therapist and prescriber have access to current information, minimizing the risk of errors and enhancing treatment continuity.

In navigating the intersection of pharmacological interventions and therapy, therapists have the opportunity to advocate for the client's voice. As they embed the client's preferences, priorities, and insights into the dialogue with prescribers, they ensure that the client remains the focal point of all decisions made.

Lastly, it's worth remembering that ultimately the goal of collaboration between therapists and prescribers is to provide a scaffold of integrated support around the individual. It's in the weaving together of expertise and compassion that we can offer a tapestry of healing—strengthened by each thread of professional input—that truly envelops and uplifts our clients.

When we, as therapists, approach our relationship with prescribers as a partnership in pursuit of a common mission, we set the stage for a more synchronized and impactful intervention. As we journey towards the shared horizon of reclaiming lives from the shadow of trauma, let us remember the power of united efforts, the hope they entail, and the promise of restoration they hold for those we serve.

Understanding the Benefits and Risks of Pharmacotherapy

As we delve into the complex and sensitive realm of trauma treatment, we recognize pharmacotherapy as a crucial tool in our kit—one capable of alleviating debilitating symptoms that obstruct the path to recovery. Pharmacological interventions can be profoundly transformative, particularly when wielded thoughtfully and in tandem with other therapeutic modalities.

Let's embark on exploring the benefits of pharmacotherapy. At its best, medication offers a reduction of overwhelming symptoms, such as anxiety, depression, and other stress-related disorders that are frequently companions of trauma. The judicious use of anti-depressants, mood stabilizers, or anti-anxiety medications, for instance, can not only improve daily functioning but also provide the emotional stability needed to actively engage in psychotherapy.

Medication can serve as a bridge over tumultuous waters, allowing individuals to access therapeutic work that might otherwise be too painful or challenging. Imagine a person so consumed by PTSD symptoms that they can't leave their home or engage in conversation. The right medication could reduce these barriers, rendering the therapeutic process accessible and fruitful.

Cognitive functions, often impaired by trauma, can also benefit from pharmacological interventions. Certain medications aid in dampening the noise of intrusive thoughts, facilitating clearer thinking and improving concentration, which is essential for cognitive-behavioral techniques employed during therapy.

Furthermore, we must consider those whose biological predispositions may render them more susceptible to intense and persistent symptoms. In these cases, pharmacotherapy may be indispensable, adjusting the body's chemical imbalances that therapy alone might not address.

However, as we navigate these waters, we must be acutely aware of the treacherous undercurrents—the risks and side effects associated with psychiatric medications. Side effects can range from mild (such as dry mouth or mild nausea) to severe (including weight gain, sexual dysfunction, or increased suicidal ideation), and they can significantly impact a person's quality of life and willingness to continue treatment.

Moreover, the complexities of trauma mean that each individual's response to medication can be highly unpredictable. What offers relief to one may exacerbate symptoms for another. This unpredictability necessitates a close collaborative relationship with psychiatrists to tailor pharmacological strategies to each person's unique biochemistry.

The risk of dependency and withdrawal is another critical consideration. Benzodiazepines, often prescribed for their rapid relief of acute anxiety, carry a high risk of dependency. Long-term use can lead to tolerance, wherein the individual requires higher doses to achieve the same therapeutic effect, thereby increasing the difficulty of discontinuation.

Medication can also sometimes mask underlying issues rather than address them directly. It's akin to applying a bandage over a deep wound without properly cleaning it; infection can lurk beneath the surface. While medication mitigates symptoms, the trauma itself remains untouched, and symptoms may resurface when medication is discontinued.

Dosage and timing also pose challenges. Finding the optimal dose—one that offers the maximum benefit with minimal side effects—is an exercise in patience and precision. And for many psychiatric medications, therapeutic effects are not immediate. Individuals must often wait weeks to assess the full impact, enduring potential side effects without immediate relief.

An additional layer comes with polypharmacy—the use of multiple medications. This practice is common in treating complex trauma cases where multiple symptoms may be present. Yet, the interactions between different medications can introduce a raft of new side effects and complications, turning the pursuit of relief into a labyrinthine task.

It's also paramount to consider the implications of abrupt discontinuation, which can lead to withdrawal symptoms or the rapid reemergence of the initial trauma-related symptoms. Hence, any decision to stop a medication must be carefully considered and meticulously planned.

Finally, we turn our gaze to the risk of medicalizing trauma. While medication can be immensely helpful, it is not a panacea. We must hold space for the reality that trauma is not solely a medical issue but one intrinsically tied to psychological, social, and environmental factors. The stories behind the symptoms need to be heard and healed, and medication should support, not overshadow, this process.

In conclusion, the intersection of pharmacotherapy and trauma care is laden with potential and pitfalls. The balance between the benefits and risks must be carefully weighed, always with the individual's well-being at the forefront. As mental health professionals, we serve as guides, empowering those we support to understand the choices before them, to find hope in healing, and to reach a place of resilience and strength.

Let us not forget that while medication can be a powerful ally, it is the human connection, understanding, and support that ultimately mend the fissures trauma has carved into lives. Pharmacotherapy, when integrated within a comprehensive, trauma-informed therapeutic approach, can truly enhance the journey toward wellness and inner peace.

Chapter 11:
Self-Care for Therapists

As we transition from exploring the multi-faceted approaches to trauma therapy and the critical collaboration with psychiatrists, it's imperative to shine a light on the healers themselves. Within Chapter 11, the essential practice of self-care for therapists takes center stage. Entering the therapeutic space, practitioners carry not only their expertise but also their humanity, a duality that requires nurturing to sustain longevity in the field. This chapter delves into the crucial understanding that therapists, while adept at facilitating healing, also encounter the emotional resonance of their clients' traumatic narratives. Embracing self-care isn't merely a recommendation; it's the scaffolding that supports the therapist's well-being and bolsters their capacity to be present and efficacious. Here, we examine the importance of recognizing symptoms of vicarious traumatization, impart strategies to foster professional health, and highlight the tools necessary to construct a resilient foundation, enabling you to continue the indispensable work of guiding others towards recovery without compromising your serenity and vitality.

Recognizing Vicarious Traumatization

Vicarious traumatization, also sometimes referred to as secondary traumatic stress, is a reality that many mental health professionals confront within the contours of their work. The impact of absorbing the traumatic stories and emotional distress of your clients can insidiously mirror the symptoms of their clients' trauma. This

115

phenomenon can affect you deeply, both professionally and personally. It's a testament to the human connection, the empathy that sits at the very heart of your therapeutic practice - but without adequate self-care, it can become a vulnerability.

Understanding this construct requires introspection and a willingness to acknowledge vulnerability. Therapists are, after all, human, inescapably susceptible to the suffering of those they seek to help. Over time, if left unchecked, therapists may find their worldviews shifting, perhaps perceiving the world through a darker lens, more chaotic, dangerous, or hopeless, a consequence echoing their clients' traumatic experiences.

Recognizing the signs of vicarious traumatization is paramount; they can be subtle or overt. They may manifest as intrusive thoughts, pervasive sadness, or feelings of being overwhelmed. Perhaps your sleep is disturbed by vivid dreams or insomnia, or maybe you find yourself disconnected from your emotions - an atypical numbness or irritability taking hold.

Physical symptoms, too, can serve as indicators - a tightness in your chest, a persistent fatigue, or even an increase in physical ailments. The toll on your mental health could also present as cognitive changes, difficulty concentrating, or reduced professional efficacy. Pay attention to these signs within yourself. They're not merely fleeting stressors; they're signposts, signaling a need for self-care and adjustment in your professional practice.

One of the first steps to combat vicarious traumatization is maintaining professional boundaries. It's easy to blur the lines, to carry your clients' burdens home, pondering their pain in silent solidarity. But recall, your role is to facilitate healing, not to bear the weight of their trauma upon your shoulders. Boundaries safeguard not only your clients but also yourself, marking the line where your professional contribution ends, and personal life begins.

Additionally, fostering self-awareness is crucial. It requires regular self-reflection, perhaps through journaling or supervision, to discern the impacts your profession has on your psyche. Cultivate this skill - it will act as both shield and compass, guiding and protecting you.

Another protective measure is building a strong support network. Colleagues, supervisors, and mentors can be invaluable, but so can connection with those outside the field. Diverse relationships foster balance, offering alternative perspectives and solace away from the intensities of therapy.

Self-care strategies are incredibly diverse, but they share a common aim: to replenish the well from which you give so much. Engage in activities that rejuvenate your spirit. Whether it's through exercise, creativity, mindfulness, or simply nature, restoring your equilibrium is not indulgent; it's essential.

Professional development is also an essential element in recognizing and managing vicarious traumatization. Continued learning about trauma, its effects, and effective coping strategies can provide you with the tools and knowledge necessary to safeguard your wellbeing.

Practicing mindfulness and meditation provide strategies for grounding and centering oneself amidst the turmoil that can accompany trauma work. They arm you with the ability to stay present with discomfort, acknowledging it but not letting it dominate your experience.

Therapy, for the therapist, should never be off the table. Personal therapy is a proactive measure, ensuring that you process your own emotional responses rather than bottling them up. It's a confidential space to explore and understand the emotional echoes of your work, away from the roles you fulfill for others.

Remember to celebrate your successes, both large and small. The nature of your work often focuses on pain and suffering, but therein also lays triumph, resilience, and healing. Recognize and honor these moments, for they are the heart of why you do what you do.

Finally, knowing when to step back is both an act of courage and wisdom. There will be times when the most professional decision you can make is to take a hiatus, to recalibrate and nurture your own mental health. This isn't defeat, it's a strategic retreat, ensuring that you can return to your practice energized and with renewed perspective.

Vicarious traumatization is not a sign of weakness, nor is it an indication of professional inadequacy. It's a natural response to the work heartfully undertaken by those brave enough to stand in the therapeutic space with those who suffer. Recognizing it is the first step. Actively addressing it is an ongoing process—one that is as vital as any other aspect of your professional practice.

Strategies for Maintaining Professional Health

As mental health professionals, we're not immune to the toll that continuous exposure to traumatic stories can take on our own well-being. It's crucial to have strategies in place to maintain our professional health and ensure the longevity of our careers. In this section, we'll explore ways to sustain and nurture your professional vitality.

Firstly, it's vital to establish strong personal boundaries. It's tempting to overextend yourself, but knowing your limits and when to say no is essential. Respect your time and energy as you do for your clients. Setting boundaries can prevent feelings of being overwhelmed and protect against the encroachment of work into personal life.

Self-awareness is a key component of professional health. Regular self-reflection on how your work impacts your emotions and thoughts will help you detect early signs of compassion fatigue. Keeping a reflective journal can be a transformative practice for monitoring your inner world.

Professional supervision is not just a requirement but a sanctuary for clinicians. Engaging in regular supervision provides an opportunity to process complex cases, share burdens, and receive valuable feedback. Embrace supervision as a space where you can be vulnerable and seek guidance.

Creating a professional support network is also essential. Building relationships with peers who understand the unique challenges of trauma therapy provides you with a sense of camaraderie and mutual support. Networking events, professional associations, and online forums are great places to start.

Emphasizing work-life balance is not a cliché; it's a critical practice. Invest in your hobbies, spend time with loved ones, and make room for rest. These activities are not just downtime; they're integral to rejuvenating your passion and energy for your work.

Prioritize physical health as you would for your clients. Regular exercise, adequate sleep, and nutritious meals are foundational to mental and physical stamina. Incorporating mindfulness or yoga can also help in maintaining a mind-body balance.

Continuing education is another important factor. Learning new techniques and gaining knowledge not only improves your practice but also keeps you engaged and intellectually stimulated. Attend workshops, read the latest research, and stay curious.

Maintaining a practice of gratitude can transform your outlook on work. Each day, take a moment to reflect on what you appreciate about your job. Gratitude can increase resilience and create a buffer against the adverse effects of stress.

Remember to celebrate your successes, no matter how small. Acknowledging the positive impact you make in your clients' lives reinforces your purpose and can provide a powerful antidote to burnout.

In addition to these practices, it's essential to develop a personal wellness plan. Be proactive and outline strategies to counteract stress and burnout. Your plan might include regular therapy for yourself, vacations, retreats or periodically assessing your career goals and alignment with personal values.

Don't underestimate the power of laughter and play. Humor can be a potent stress-reliever, and allowing yourself to be playful can bring joy and lightness into your life. Incorporate aspects of play into your daily routine to keep your spirit uplifted.

Lastly, practice self-compassion. Treat yourself with the same kindness and understanding that you offer your clients. It's okay to experience difficult emotions; what's important is how you tend to them. Self-compassion fosters resilience and compassion towards others.

By integrating these strategies into your professional practice, you create a sustainable career that not only serves your clients but also respects and honors your own professional health. It's this dedication to balance that enables you to be a beacon of hope for those you serve.

Incorporating these strategies into daily life requires effort and commitment, yet the rewards are manifold. As you continue to invest in your professional health, you'll find yourself better equipped to meet the challenges of trauma therapy with strength and grace. Remember, your health is the foundation upon which your ability to help others rests, and preserving it is one of the most significant contributions you can make to the field of trauma-informed therapy.

Building Resilience and Preventing Burnout

As therapists, you give immeasurably to your clients. Yet, to nurture their journey towards healing, it's vital that you first look after your well-being. It is only from a replenished well that one can continue to offer the elixir of empathy and understanding that trauma work requires. Building resilience and preventing burnout isn't just beneficial; it's imperative for the sustainability of your practice.

Resilience, the ability to bounce back from challenges, is like a muscle that can be strengthened with proper care. Consistent self-care practices can bolster your resilience, equipping you to manage the emotional demands of trauma therapy. These practices can and should be as varied and unique as you are, encompassing physical, emotional, and spiritual components to support your holistic health.

Self-awareness is the foundation of building resilience. By cultivating a keen understanding of your responses to stress, you can identify early signs of fatigue and respond proactively. Mindfulness techniques are invaluable tools for developing this self-awareness, enabling you to stay present and engaged both within yourself and with your clients.

Physical self-care is crucial and often overlooked in the mental health field. Regular exercise, quality sleep, and nutritious eating habits aren't luxuries—they are the bedrock of cognitive function and emotional stability. They keep your body ready to face the rigors of trauma work with strength and vitality.

Establishing clear boundaries is another key aspect of maintaining professional health. Being able to delineate where your professional role starts and ends can prevent the blurring of lines that often leads to emotional fatigue. Remember, saying 'no' or 'not now' can be a profound act of self-care.

Connection with colleagues offers a vital support network. Supervision, peer groups, and professional communities can serve as a sanctuary for sharing experiences, relieving stresses, and fostering a shared understanding of the unique demands of your work. Do not underestimate the power of being heard and understood by those who walk a similar path.

Regular breaks and vacations are not indulgent—they are necessary intervals that allow you to come back to your work with fresh eyes and renewed energy. Intentional rest is as important as the work itself, offering you space to recharge and reflect.

Engaging in reflective practice is another method of fostering resilience. Writing journals or engaging in supervision allows you to process the emotional resonance of the work you do. Reflection helps in distilling experiences, integrating lessons learned, and developing strategies for personal growth.

Mental detaching from work is essential when you're off the clock. Cultivate hobbies, interests, and activities that bring you joy and relaxation. They will act as a counterbalance to the heavacity of your professional life, allowing you to return with a sense of wholeness.

Formal resilience training can also be beneficial. Workshops and courses designed to enhance coping skills can provide new strategies and perspectives that contribute to your personal growundth as a compassionate clinician.

Practicing gratitude can shift your focus from the burdens of trauma work to the profound privilege of assisting others in their healing journey. A daily gratitude practice, whether through journaling or mindful reflection, can nurture an attitude that cherishes the positive aspects of your life and work.

Attend to your spiritual or philosophical needs, as they can provide a sense of purpose and perspective. Whether through meditation, prayer, or engaging with nature, attending to your spirit is as vital to resilience as addressing your physiological and psychological needs. There is nourishment found in a purpose that transcends the day-to-day.

Finally, never hesitate to seek therapy for yourself. We can't provide a healing space for others if we are neglecting our wounds. Therapy is an act of self-care that validates your experiences and provides strategies to cope with the unique stressors of the profession.

Incorporating creativity into your routine can offer a restorative outlet for your emotions. Creative expression, be it through art, music, dance, or writing, enables you to process and release the emotional residue that comes with trauma therapy. It's a pathway to discovering joy and vibrancy amidst the seriousness of your work.

By integrating these practices of self-care into your life, you can build a resilience that not only sustains you but also enriches the therapeutic space you provide for your clients. Resilience isn't just about survival; it's about thriving in the midst of challenges and emerging stronger, wiser, and more compassionate. As you guide others through the wilderness of their trauma, remember to tend to your own well-being with as much dedication and kindness. Your ability to do so doesn't just make you a better therapist; it makes you an exemplar of the healing you aim to facilitate.

Chapter 12:
Advances and Future Directions
in Trauma Therapy

As we turn the page from understanding the impacts and interventions associated with trauma, we find ourselves gazing toward the horizon of **advances and future directions in trauma therapy**. Empowering those we serve with innovative, research-backed methodologies is paramount—as such, the ongoing pursuit of *knowledge evolution* and the **embrace of technology** represent the new vanguard in trauma treatment. With data-driven discoveries illuminating once-shadowed pathways, professionals across the mental health spectrum are witnessing a renaissance in therapeutic practices. The integration of technology-assisted therapies is not just a glimpse into the future, but a reality unfurling before us, offering unprecedented avenues for connection, assessment, and healing. Moreover, we're called to stand ever vigilant and proactive as advocates, influencing policy and systematic change for a society deeply attuned to the needs of those healing from trauma. The journey ahead is one of both promise and profound responsibility—a challenge to which we must rise with courage and a steadfast commitment to progress and authenticity in our practice.

Innovations in Trauma Therapy Research

The landscape of trauma therapy research is ever-evolving, with innovative techniques and methodologies continually emerging. As we delve further into this robust area of study, we find at the heart of it all one unwavering purpose: to transcend the boundaries of our current knowledge and provide those who have been touched by trauma the keys to unlock their healing potential.

One burgeoning area of research is the exploration of neuro-plasticity within trauma recovery. The malleability of the brain suggests that it can redefine and rewire itself following traumatic experiences. This framework bolsters the efficacy of therapies aimed at altering negative thought patterns and enhancing mental flexibility. Studies are progressively honing in on how specific therapeutic approaches can intentionally shape the brain's neural pathways, potentially leading to lasting changes in emotional processing and behavior.

Further, the integration of genetic and epigenetic research into the therapy process is shedding light on how trauma affects genetic expression. Investigators are focusing on identifying biomarkers that can predict and improve treatment outcomes—a transformational shift that could lead to personalized treatment plans that respect the unique physiological makeup of each individual.

Another promising innovation involves the augmentation of traditional psychotherapy with psychopharmacological treatments. The quest to uncover how medications can best support psycho-therapeutic techniques is gaining momentum as research explores the synergistic potential between medication and mindfulness practices, somatic therapies, and cognitive interventions.

Further, as our world becomes progressively digital, virtual and augmented reality tools are being welcomed into the therapist's toolkit. By incorporating these technologies, researchers are exploring how they can create controlled environments to safely expose individuals to traumatic stimuli and reinforce coping strategies in a highly immersive manner.

As trauma therapy methodologies become more sophisticated, so do the assessment tools at our disposal. Data analytics and machine learning are beginning to offer groundbreaking ways to parse the complex variables of trauma exposure and response. Being able to more accurately predict treatment courses based on expansive datasets can enhance therapeutic precision and effectiveness.

Moreover, the attention given to the gut-brain axis and its influence on emotional well-being offers a fresh lens through which to examine trauma therapy. Advocates of this research are examining how nutrition, probiotics, and other gut-targeted interventions can contribute to improved mental health outcomes in trauma survivors.

The importance of sleep in trauma processing and recovery is another rich area of study. Researchers are now unpacking the intricate relationship between trauma, sleep disturbances, and recovery modalities. Innovative therapies that seek to restore healthful sleep patterns are currently being tested and integrated into holistic treatment models.

Not to be overlooked is the emerging recognition of the healing potential within mindfulness and meditation practices. Investigators are continually identifying the active components of these practices that contribute to trauma recovery and how they can be systematically introduced into treatment plans.

Artificial intelligence is also beginning to insinuate itself into the therapeutic context. By employing algorithms that tailor treatments to individual needs or even assist in diagnosing PTSD and other trauma-related conditions, AI has the potential to revolutionize the way we approach therapy.

Furthermore, the study of resilience factors following trauma exposure is expanding. Instead of solely focusing on the aftereffects of trauma, research is shifting towards understanding what allows individuals to thrive post-trauma. Identifying and nurturing these resilience factors could empower survivors and refocus therapy on growth and development.

One can't overlook the groundbreaking advances made through societal and cultural research in trauma therapy. By investigating the role of sociocultural factors, researchers hope to craft interventions that are fine-tuned to the nuanced experiences of diverse populations, including those historically underrepresented in trauma research.

Lastly, there is an invigorated pursuit of the impact that animal-assisted therapies have on healing trauma. By understanding the bond between humans and animals, researchers are identifying another potential avenue to facilitate connection, trust, and emotional recovery for those with trauma histories.

The research frontier in trauma therapy is vast and replete with promise. With relentless curiosity, researchers and practitioners work side by side to turn the unknown into groundbreaking therapeutic approaches. Each innovation embodies the commitment to those whose lives we seek to uplift, echoing a message of actualizable hope and renewal.

As we continue to push the boundaries of possibility, let us remain steadfast in our dedication to this noble cause. Together, with every study, with every clinical trial, with every enlightened moment shared with a survivor—let us illuminate the path toward growth, healing, and the reclamation of empowerment for all who walk the journey of trauma recovery.

Technology-Assisted Therapies

In an era where technological advancements have permeated nearly every aspect of life, the field of trauma therapy is no exception. Technology-assisted therapies (TAT) have emerged as a formidable complement to traditional therapeutic approaches, offering unique avenues for addressing the deeply rooted impacts of trauma. Harnessing technology in therapy can pave the way for innovative treatment modalities that can transform the therapeutic landscape and open up new possibilities for healing.

At the forefront of TAT is the use of virtual reality (VR). VR technology immerses clients in environments where they can safely confront and work through traumatic memories, all under the careful guidance of a clinician. This method extends beyond traditional talk therapy by offering a controlled, but lifelike, experience where individuals can learn to process and cope with traumatic events in real time. The immersive nature of VR therapy has shown promise, particularly for those who have found traditional exposure therapies challenging.

An innovative aspect of TAT is the development of mobile health applications, known as mHealth. These applications can serve as both therapeutic tools and as a means of monitoring client progress in real-time. For clients, mHealth apps can provide reinforcement of skills learned in therapy sessions through interactive activities, reminders for self-care, and mood tracking features. For therapists, these digital tools offer insights into the client's progress outside of sessions, allowing for more personalized and responsive care.

Artificial intelligence (AI) and machine learning are being integrated into trauma therapy to offer more personalized treatment plans. AI algorithms can analyze client data to identify patterns and predict outcomes, which can aid therapists in making more precise and timely interventions. Furthermore, chatbots and virtual assistants equipped with AI can provide immediate support to clients, offering coping strategies and crisis intervention when human support may not be immediately available.

Teletherapy, the delivery of therapeutic services via telecommunication technologies, has exploded in popularity, particularly in the wake of global crises that necessitate physical distancing. This format has been essential in ensuring continuity of care and has made trauma therapy accessible to individuals who may not have been able to receive in-person therapy due to geographical, physical, or social barriers.

Biofeedback and neurofeedback are also gaining traction in the TAT sphere. When integrating these technologies, therapists can help clients gain greater control over physiological responses that are often dysregulated due to trauma, such as heart rate variability and brain wave activity. By learning to influence these responses through visual or auditory feedback, clients can develop a more robust set of coping mechanisms to mitigate the effects of trauma on the body and mind.

Online support groups have multiplied, offering individuals the chance to connect with others on the healing journey, fostering community, and collective resilience. These platforms can bridge the gap between individual therapy sessions and provide a sense of belonging, which is particularly potent for those who have experienced trauma that led to social isolation or marginalization.

Gaming technology, though often overlooked, has found a place in trauma therapy as well. Therapeutic video games are being developed to help individuals with trauma-related symptoms. These games incorporate evidence-based therapeutic concepts in a format that is engaging and motivating, contributing to resilience and problem-solving skills.

Another emerging area of interest is the application of augmented reality (AR) in trauma therapy. Different from VR, AR overlays digital information onto the real world and can be used to create "safe spaces" for clients or to externalize inner experiences in a tangible way, complementing therapeutic processes like imaginal exposure and cognitive restructuring.

Information and communication technologies have also advanced the reach and efficiency of psychoeducation. With trauma-informed educational platforms and resources being available online, clients can deepen their understanding of trauma and its effects, which is an essential component of the healing process. Educated clients are empowered clients, capable of actively participating in their recovery journey.

Despite the promising potential of TAT, ethical considerations must be accounted for. Confidentiality, privacy, and informed consent are paramount when integrating technology into therapy. The digital divide and disparities in access to technology must also be addressed to prevent the inadvertent exclusion of certain populations from benefiting from these innovative tools.

Research into the efficacy of TAT is continually evolving, and its widespread acceptance will depend on ongoing validation and the empirical support of these methods. As we look to the future, it is imperative that professionals in the field stay abreast of the latest research findings, ensuring that technology-assisted interventions are both evidence-based and implemented with the highest therapeutic standards.

Training and competence in the use of TAT are also of vital importance. As mental health professionals, we must commit to learning about these new technologies, understanding their capabilities and limitations, and acquiring the skills necessary to integrate them effectively into our practices.

In conclusion, technology-assisted therapies offer exciting new pathways for those affected by trauma to explore healing. As we continue to embrace these advancements, we must do so with a balanced perspective, combining innovation with the wisdom of traditional therapeutic techniques that have stood the test of time. In harmonizing these approaches, we expand the horizons of possibility for our clients and for the field of trauma therapy.

Lastly, let us remember that technology, while a powerful tool, is an adjunct to, and not a replacement for, the human connection that lies at the heart of the therapeutic alliance. It is our empathy, presence, and unwavering belief in the resilience of the human spirit that remain central to guiding our clients toward growth and healing, with technology as our ally on this transformative journey.

Policy and Advocacy for Trauma-Informed Care

Trauma-informed care represents not just a shift in individual practice but a transformative movement that necessitates robust policies and advocacy efforts. This fundamental change in societal attitudes and professional norms has the potential to generate pervasive improvements in the way trauma survivors are understood and supported.

To truly adopt a trauma-informed mindset, we must tirelessly advocate for policies that recognize the widespread impact of trauma. This involves pushing for legislation that supports trauma-informed education for professionals across various sectors, including healthcare, social services, education, and the legal system. Working in concert, these fields can provide a more cohesive and supportive framework for individuals affected by trauma.

Crucial to our advocacy efforts is the need to secure funding for trauma research and trauma-informed services. Resources must be dedicated to not only understanding the nuances of trauma but also to implementing practices that have been demonstrated to help heal and empower those who have been impacted. Mental health professionals are positioned to lead these initiatives by lending their expertise to guide effective policy development.

Furthermore, it is imperative to strive for policies that foster accessibility and inclusivity. Trauma therapy should not be a privilege restricted to a few but a readily available service for all who need it, regardless of socioeconomic status, race, ethnicity, or gender. Advocating for sliding-scale fees, insurance coverage, and grants can help bridge this gap and bring healing within reach for diverse populations.

In addition, we must emphasize the importance of trauma-informed practices within institutions, such as schools and workplaces. By integrating understanding and flexibility into these environments, we can create safe spaces that recognize and adapt to the needs of trauma survivors. Campaigning for trauma-informed training programs in these areas can help build a community that is sensitive to the echoes of trauma.

One cannot underestimate the power of partnerships and coalitions in the realm of advocacy. Aligning with other organizations, advocacy groups, and trauma survivors themselves can amplify our efforts and bring about significant change. These partnerships can also facilitate the sharing of knowledge and best practices, further strengthening the case for trauma-informed approaches.

To this end, mental health professionals can engage in educational outreach, participating in public speaking, writing articles, and joining advisory boards to promote awareness about trauma and its pervasive effects. Becoming thought leaders in this field can shape public opinion and influence decision-makers.

Monitoring and influencing policy implementation is equally important. Advocates need to ensure that laws and regulations are not only written but enacted in ways that truly benefit trauma survivors. This could involve participating in task forces or committees that oversee the execution of trauma-informed initiatives.

In the spirit of empowerment central to trauma-informed care, advocates should encourage the voices of trauma survivors themselves. Involving individuals in the shaping of policies and programs ensures that their real needs and experiences are not just represented but are also front and center in driving change.

Educational systems also play a vital role in fostering a trauma-informed future. Collaborating with universities and training programs to include trauma-informed curriculum can equip new generations of professionals with the skills and knowledge required to support and treat trauma effectively.

Measuring the impact of advocacy efforts is critical for continual improvement and justification of policies. Building a body of evidence that demonstrates the effectiveness of trauma-informed practices can substantiate the need for ongoing support and resources.

There's also an ethical imperative in advocacy. Mental health professionals must ensure that the policies for which they advocate uphold the highest ethical standards, protecting client confidentiality, and respecting the autonomy and dignity of all individuals. This ethical compass should guide all endeavors within the realm of policy and advocacy.

Lastly, sustainable advocacy encompasses self-care for advocates themselves. The work of an advocate can be trying, requiring resilience and emotional fortitude. Prioritizing one's own well-being is paramount to maintain the energy and commitment needed to fuel long-term advocacy efforts.

As we strive to shape a future in trauma therapy, being an advocate for trauma-informed care is not an optional extra—it's an indispensable part of our duty as mental health professionals. Through deliberate, informed, and compassionate advocacy, we can lay the groundwork for a society better equipped to heal, support, and empower trauma survivors. It is in this way that our collective efforts will emit a beacon of hope that signals a brighter, more understanding future.

Online Review Request for this Book

As we navigate the evolving landscape of trauma therapy together, your insights and experiences are invaluable; if this book has enhanced your understanding or practice, I encourage you to share your thoughts online to empower others in our community to foster resilience and healing in those they serve.

Chapter 13:
A Beacon of Hope – The Path
Forward in Trauma Therapy

In our journey through understanding and treating trauma, we've uncovered the depths of human resilience and the profound capacity for renewal. Together, we've traversed the complex landscapes of the mind and body, recognizing the intricate interplay between our neurological wiring and the stories etched into our being. As we stand on the precipice of this journey, let's consider the path forward.

The field of trauma therapy is ever-evolving, and as practitioners, our mission is to evolve with it. With the foundation of trauma-informed care principles, we have a robust scaffolding upon which we can build more compassionate, effective treatment strategies. We're tasked to be stewards of hope, guiding individuals as they transform their pain into empowerment, and their wounds into wellsprings of strength.

Healing from trauma isn't a linear process, nor is it one-size-fits-all. Our exploration of various therapies—from cognitive-behavioral interventions to somatic approaches—highlights the necessity for personalization in treatment plans. Prolonged Exposure, EMDR, and DBT may hold keys for some, while others find solace in narrative and expressive therapies. It's our role to tailor these keys to unlock each individual's doors to recovery.

The therapeutic relationship remains a beacon itself—a safe harbor where trust is the currency and validation is the compass. Creating environments of empowerment matters more now than ever. We, as therapists, need to embody these values consistently to fortify the walls within which healing can occur.

As we move into the future, we must continue to prioritize culturally sensitive assessment techniques, ensuring that our therapy rooms are inclusive spaces where diversity is not just acknowledged but celebrated. The depths of understanding we've developed about the impact of trauma on marginalized groups demand action. Let's pave the way for these insights to inform policies and advocacy efforts that extend far beyond our offices.

It's crucial to acknowledge the special populations that carry unique burdens of trauma. From the tender psyches of children to the often-overlooked trauma in older adults, these individuals remind us why we must adapt and refine our methods. Just as trauma presents itself in myriad forms, so too must our therapies be numerous and malleable.

Let's also cast a light on the importance of collaboration within our field and with the wider circles of healthcare professionals. The marriage of pharmacological interventions and psychotherapy exemplifies the holistic approach necessary for treating the multi-dimensional aspect of trauma. Building bridges with colleagues in psychiatry and other disciplines enriches our treatment models and, ultimately, improves patient outcomes.

Reflection on self-care for therapists is more than a chapter in a text; it's a daily practice. Let's commit to safeguarding our well-being as fervently as we do for those we serve. Recognizing the signs of vicarious traumatization, fostering resilience, and preventing burnout aren't just professional responsibilities—they're anchors that keep us grounded and able to serve effectively.

Advances in technology-assisted therapies and innovative research beckon us toward new frontiers. We're poised to harness these advancements, integrating cutting-edge tools and evidence-based practices with the timeless human elements of empathy and connection. As the terrain of trauma therapy expands, let's be pioneering explorers, keen to incorporate new findings and more nuanced understandings into our work.

At this juncture, let's take a measured view of our role. We have embraced the title of healers and educators, advocates and lifelong learners. The call to cultivate a brighter future for trauma survivors rings out with urgency and clarity. We are called to respond not merely as clinicians but as champions of the human spirit.

The path forward is not without its challenges, but it is rich with opportunity. We can navigate any adversities by anchoring ourselves in the values that have guided our journey: compassion, curiosity, flexibility, and perseverance. If we embody these, we serve not just as therapists but as beacons of hope ourselves.

As the chapters of this book come to a close, your work in the world blossoms anew. May each client you encounter feel the radiance of hope you carry. May you see the seeds of your efforts bloom into a landscape of healing. And may the path you walk be lit with the knowledge that in helping others overcome trauma, you illuminate the way for a brighter, more resilient future for all.

We stand at a precipice, looking back on the strides made and ahead to the journey that continues. It's a path etched in hope, paved in dedication, and traveled with the courage to embrace growth and change. Let us step forward with the assurance that our collective efforts will leave an indelible mark on the field of trauma therapy—a legacy of transformation and healing.

Now is the moment to reach out with an open heart and a steady hand. Let us be the agents of change, fostering recovery and resilience in a world that so desperately seeks it. For in the darkest of times, we have found that hope is not only necessary—it is vital. And it is us, as therapists, who can nurture this hope, helping it to flourish in the lives of those who come to us in their most vulnerable moments.

Appendix A:
Trauma-Informed Therapy
Resources for Practitioners

Delving into the heart of compassionate and effective trauma therapy, we recognize the need for a repository of resources that can deepen your expertise and enhance your practice. Consider this appendix as a toolbox—thoughtfully curated and neatly organized—to support your ongoing journey in facilitating healing for those who've been through deeply distressing or disturbing events.

Professional Organizations and Networks

Connecting with professional bodies provides avenues for continued education, shared knowledge, and peer support. The following are pivotal to the trauma-informed field:

- **International Society for Traumatic Stress Studies (ISTSS)**: Offers comprehensive resources including training opportunities, research updates, and an annual conference.

- **The National Child Traumatic Stress Network (NCTSN)**: Delivers resources related to the impact of trauma on children and young people, encompassing varied therapeutic modalities.

- **The American Psychological Association (APA) Trauma Division**: A platform for resources and community engagement specific to psychological trauma and treatment.

Educational Materials and Training

The pursuit of excellence in trauma-informed therapy benefits enormously from ongoing education. Check out:

- *Trauma-Informed Care in Behavioral Health Services*: A SAMHSA publication catering to behavioral health service providers.

- Continuing education courses from reputable institutions focusing on trauma-related subjects.

- Webinars, seminars, and online workshops from trauma-focused organizations.

Books and Literature

Ground your practice in wisdom and insights distilled from key texts in the field:

- **The Body Keeps the Score** by Bessel van der Kolk, a pivotal read on understanding and treating trauma.

- **Waking the Tiger** by Peter Levine, offers groundbreaking perspectives on healing trauma through somatic experiencing.

- A range of peer-reviewed journals such as *Journal of Traumatic Stress* and *Trauma, Violence, & Abuse* that serve as an excellent source of research and case studies.

Therapeutic Modalities and Techniques

Being adept with various modalities boosts your adaptability to diverse client needs:

- Explore advanced training in Eye Movement Desensitization and Reprocessing (EMDR), Somatic Experiencing (SE), and Dialectical Behavior Therapy (DBT) for trauma.

- Seek certifications or skills-based workshops in Cognitive Processing Therapy (CPT) and Prolonged Exposure Therapy (PE).

- Stay refreshed on trauma-focused CBT for children and adolescents, especially for those practicing in environments with younger clients.

Community and Peer Support

Never underestimate the power of a supportive professional community:

- Join local or online groups for trauma therapists to exchange knowledge and seek consult.

- Mentorship programs where experienced clinicians guide you in refining your approach to trauma therapy.

- Networking at conferences and local events can enrich your understanding and offer new perspectives.

Self-Care and Professional Wellness

Caring for yourself is as crucial as caring for others. Resources to support your well-being include:

- **Self-Care for the Mental Health Practitioner**, a book that provides strategies to manage stress and prevent burnout.

- Online courses and webinars focusing on self-care and resilience for therapists.

- Retreats and professional therapy services geared toward mental health professionals.

Your transformative role in guiding clients on the path to recovery is invaluable, and it's vital to remain well-equipped for the journey ahead. These resources serve to embolden your practice with a wealth of knowledge and support, enabling you to continue providing the deep-seated compassion and skilled intervention that characterizes a truly trauma-informed therapist.

Appendix B:
Assessment Tools and Measures

As we continue to unravel the layers of trauma-informed therapy, it's crucial to highlight the instruments that clinicians use to illuminate the depth of their clients' experiences. In this Appendix, we delve into an array of assessment tools and measures that serve as the compass guiding us through the oftentimes murky waters of psychological assessment.

Before we can begin to measure the imprints of trauma or navigate the turbulent seas of its impact, having a reliable set of tools is indispensable. These tools are more than mere checklists or questionnaires; they are the means through which empathy can be channeled, understanding can be deepened, and healing journeys can commence.

Importance of Selecting Suitable Assessment Instruments

Every individual's experience with trauma is as distinct as their fingerprint. Thus, the choice of assessment tools should be made with a keen eye to accuracy, cultural sensitivity, and relevance to the presenting concerns. A toolbox that's rich in diverse instruments enhances the clinician's ability to tailor the assessment process to each unique narrative.

Remember, the true strength of an assessment tool lies in its ability to resonate with the person's experience, fostering a space where their voice can be heard, and their pain acknowledged. It's a stepping stone towards empowerment and the reclaiming of their narrative.

Comprehensive Assessment Tools

When we speak of comprehensive assessment tools, we're looking at instruments that take into account the multifaceted nature of trauma. These tools often cover a broad spectrum of symptoms and allow for the nuanced understanding required to support individuals on their healing journey.

- **The Clinician-Administered PTSD Scale (CAPS)** is widely considered the gold standard in PTSD assessment. It provides a detailed measure of the frequency and intensity of symptoms and garners significant weight in both clinical and research settings.

- **The Trauma History Questionnaire (THQ)** offers insight into the breadth of traumatic events an individual has experienced, serving as a comprehensive screen for a variety of trauma types.

Targeted Symptom Measures

Targeted symptom measures allow clinicians to zero in on specific aspects of the trauma response. Through these tools, you can gain clarity about particular areas of disturbance, which is essential for crafting a finely tuned treatment plan.

- **The PTSD Checklist (PCL)** is a self-report measure that assesses the severity of PTSD symptoms related to DSM criteria.

- **The Dissociative Experiences Scale (DES)** offers an evaluation of dissociative symptoms, often prevalent in complex trauma.

Culturally Attuned and Gender-Specific Instruments

Let's not forget about the cultural and gender-specific nuances that are intrinsic to an individual's experience. Using tools that are sensitive to cultural, gender, and other demographic variables is not just best practice—it's a cornerstone of trauma-informed care.

1. **The Cultural Formulation Interview (CFI)**, included in the DSM-5, assists clinicians in exploring the impact of cultural factors on the client's experience and presentation of symptoms.

2. **The Gender-Based Violence Assessment Tools** recognize the complexities of trauma that stems from gender-based violence and the unique needs that arise from such experiences.

Clinicians must continuously refine their skills in selecting and applying the appropriate tools for each individual's assessment. These measures are powerful allies in the quest to understand and alleviate trauma's grip on the mind and body.

As we conclude this Appendix, let's embrace the profound responsibility that comes with wielding these tools. Let's use them to shine a light on the path to recovery, to chart the course for resilience, and to lovingly guide those in our care towards shores of hope and healing.

Appendix C:
Guidelines for Safe Practice and
Ethical Considerations

In the landscape of trauma therapy, practitioners are tasked with navigating a journey that is as delicate as it is profound. Guided by the principles of trauma-informed care, our mandate is not only to facilitate healing but also to safeguard the dignity and the very humanity of those we serve. Within this appendix, we delineate the guidelines for safe practice and ethical considerations, a compass by which to steer the therapeutic encounter toward a horizon of trust, respect, and integrity.

Foundational Principles of Ethical Practice

At the heart of any therapeutic engagement, especially within the realms distorted by trauma, are the ethical principles that must undergird each decision, each interaction, and every therapeutic strategy engaged. Among these principles, we hold the values of autonomy, beneficence, nonmaleficence, justice, and fidelity as our unwavering guides.

- *Autonomy:* Honor the individual's right to self-determination. This demands a deep listening to, and respect for, the client's experiences, choices, and perspectives.

- *Beneficence:* Aim to promote the well-being of clients. Every therapeutic intervention must serve the client's healing and growth.

- *Nonmaleficence:* Above all, do no harm. This necessitates an acute awareness of potential retraumatization and a commitment to avoiding it.

- *Justice:* Ensure fair and equitable treatment. Recognize and actively work against the disparities and barriers that clients may face.

- *Fidelity:* Maintain trustworthiness and reliability. This includes but isn't limited to confidentiality, honesty, and the fulfillment of commitments made to the client.

Ethical Decision-Making in Trauma Therapy

When confronted with ethical dilemmas, a practitioner's innate wisdom must be complemented by a structured approach to decision-making. This includes recognizing the dilemma, consulting ethical codes, considering relevant laws and regulations, seeking supervision or consultation, and evaluating possible courses of action for their potential impact. Documenting this process serves as both a reflective tool and a record of due diligence.

Maintaining Professional Boundaries

Boundaries are the architecture within which the therapeutic relationship develops. They must be maintained with intentionality and clarity. It's critical to recognize when a boundary is nearing breach, whether it involves touch, self-disclosure, or dual relationships, and to navigate back toward safety. Boundaries are not barriers; they are the outlines within which the sacred therapeutic space exists.

Considerations for Informed Consent

Informed consent is not a mere formality; it is an ongoing conversation, one that underpins the collaborative nature of therapy. A transparent explanation of treatment approaches, potential risks, confidentiality and its limits, as well as the client's right to withdraw consent at any time, fortifies a foundation of informed agreement and mutual respect between therapist and client.

Continued Competency and Education

The arena of trauma therapy is ever-evolving, and staying attuned to new insights, techniques, and ethical considerations is paramount to safe practice. Continuing education, peer consultation, and regular supervision ensure that the care offered reflects the growing body of knowledge and maintains its efficacy and integrity.

Cultural Sensitivity and Humility

Cultural sensitivity and humility stretch beyond an acknowledgment of diversity. They demand a practitioner's dedication to understanding and valuing the client's cultural context, mitigating biases, and adapting methods to align with the client's cultural identity and experiences.

The journey forward in trauma therapy calls for practitioners to not only bear witness to the resiliency and suffering of clients but also to constantly refine the ethical compass by which we navigate these profound depths. Anchoring ourselves in these guidelines for safe practice and ethical considerations ensures that we honor the very humanity that brings us to this work, fostering a healing alliance where trust, safety, and growth can flourish.

Scan for Other Books by the Author

www.ingramcontent.com/pod-product-compliance
Lightning Source LLC
Chambersburg PA
CBHW020438290526
45785CB00002B/902